T0144736

BASIC HEALTH PUBLICATIONS USER'S GUIDE

TO

PROTEIN AND AMINO ACIDS

Learn How Protein Foods and Their Building Blocks Can Improve Your Mood and Health.

KERI MARSHALL, M.S., N.D.

JACK CHALLEM Series Editor

The information contained in this book is based upon the research and personal and professional experiences of the author. It is not intended as a substitute for consulting with your physician or other healthcare provider. Any attempt to diagnose and treat an illness should be done under the direction of a healthcare professional.

The publisher does not advocate the use of any particular healthcare protocol but believes the information in this book should be available to the public. The publisher and author are not responsible for any adverse effects or consequences resulting from the use of the suggestions, preparations, or procedures discussed in this book. Should the reader have any questions concerning the appropriateness of any procedures or preparations mentioned, the author and the publisher strongly suggest consulting a professional healthcare advisor.

Series Editor: Jack Challem
Editor: Tara Durkin
Typesetter: Gary A. Rosenberg
Series Cover Designer: Mike Stromberg

Basic Health Publications User's Guides are published by Basic Health Publications, Inc.

ISBN: 978-1-59120-157-1 (Pbk.)
ISBN: 978-1-68162-871-4 (Hardcover)

CONTENTS

INTRODUCTION

It seems hard to believe that protein—a nutrient absolutely essential for life—has become controversial. This User's Guide demystifies protein and explains its many health benefits, as well as the importance of supplemental amino acids, which are the individual building blocks of protein.

Next to water, protein is the most abundant substance in the body. Approximately 20 percent of total body weight is made up of protein. Skin, hair, nails, muscles, eyes, and internal organs such as the heart and brain are largely made of protein.

Dietary protein is absolutely essential for growth and development of the human body. A diet absent in protein leads to malnutrition and ultimately death. As you can see, protein is an essential part of nutrition, as well as a primary component of the body's composition.

Proteins play a critical role in virtually every physiological and biochemical process in the body. Proteins serve as cell communicators through the action of neurotransmitters. They are also essential for blood clotting, immune system development, and formation of milk during lactation.

A balanced diet should provide sufficient amounts of high-quality protein from a variety of sources. All proteins are not the same. For example, vegetable-based proteins provide different properties than animal-based proteins.

Between the pages of the *User's Guide to Pro-*

tein and Amino Acids you will learn all about amino acids. You will discover how a particular sequence of amino acids strung together determines the unique qualities of a protein. Certain amino acids can be found in high amounts in some proteins, while they are absent in other proteins.

Any discussion of protein would not be complete without a discussion of the many diets being promoted today that are based on dietary protein intake. "Fewer carbohydrates, more protein" seems to be all we hear lately with regard to dieting. Is this the best advice?

The *User's Guide to Protein and Amino Acids* explores different diets that are popular today. Fact is separated from fad regarding both high- and low-protein diets. You should walk away from this book with an understanding of how some diets are beneficial for short-term, rapid weight loss, while others are ideal for weight maintenance.

In the following chapters you will begin to understand the complex nature of proteins and the impact of protein intake on body weight and overall health. In addition, this User's Guide will discuss the therapeutic benefits of different protein supplements, as well as individual amino acid supplements.

CHAPTER 1

WHAT IS
A PROTEIN?

Protein was the first substance to be recognized as an essential part of health. The name "protein" was derived from the Greek word meaning "of first importance."

Proteins, like carbohydrates and fats, are considered to be organic matter because they are made up of carbon, oxygen, and hydrogen molecules. These molecules, in combination, are responsible for the living tissues of plants and animals. Proteins are unique in that, unlike carbohydrates and fats, they are also made up of a nitrogen molecule.

"Amino acid" is the name given to the basic structural unit of proteins. Nitrogen molecules are combined with hydrogen molecules to make what is called an amino group (see Figure 1). Each amino acid also has a carboxyl group, which is made up of carbon, oxygen, and hydrogen. Amino acids have what is called an "R" group, which is a side group that distinguishes one amino acid from another.

Amino groups and carboxyl groups are not chemically reactive. Essentially, they are the stable part of an amino acid. The side group is what characterizes an amino acid and ultimately decides its fate. Amino acids can be charged or uncharged, acidic or basic.

To date, more than 300 amino acids have been described in nature. Of the 300, only 20 are commonly found in mammals.

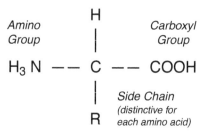

Figure 1. Amino Group

WHERE DOES PROTEIN COME FROM?

Protein is one of three available energy sources found in food. Fats and carbohydrates also provide the body with energy from food. When food is ingested, the body is able to metabolically convert a usable form of energy called a calorie. Per gram of protein ingested, the body is able to manufacture 4.0 calories. For carbohydrates, 1 gram is also equivalent to 4.0 calories. One gram of fat, on the other hand, is equivalent to 9.0 calories.

ENERGY DERIVED FROM FOOD	
1 gram	**Calories**
Protein	4.0
Carbohydrates	4.0
Fat	9.0

Foods high in protein are complete proteins in that they have sufficient quantity and variation of all twenty amino acids. Examples of complete proteins are animal-based foods such as fish, poultry, beef, pork, and wild game. Eggs and dairy products also have sufficient amino acid composition and are considered complete.

NITROGEN: WHERE DOES IT COME FROM AND WHERE DOES IT GO?

Plants make protein from nitrogen that is

obtained from ammonia and nitrates found in soil. Some plants, such as legumes, have the ability to extract nitrogen from bacteria in the atmosphere surrounding it. Animals obtain their nitrogen from eating plants and animals. When a plant or animal dies, the nitrogen in its fleshy tissue decomposes and nitrogen is returned to the soil.

THE QUALITY OF PROTEIN

Protein foods have been classified according to the body's ability to digest and utilize them. The measurement of how efficiently our bodies utilize protein is called *net protein utilization (NPU)*. This number is determined by the ratio of weight gained by a person on a particular protein to the weight that person gains on casein, a known high-quality protein derived from cow's milk. This number is based upon the assumption that weight gain is proportional to the gain in body protein. This method determines whether or not a protein source has all twenty amino acids and in correct ratios.

NPU

Net protein utilization; tells us how efficiently our bodies use a particular protein source.

Eggs from chicken are considered to have the highest NPU. After eggs, in descending order, are fish, cow's milk and cheese, brown rice, red meat, and poultry. It is important to understand that this number is not based on actual grams of protein but on how efficiently the body utilizes these grams. Brown rice, while high on the NPU list, is not a complete protein; that is, it does not contain all twenty amino acids. Eggs are highest on this scale because they have as close to a perfect amino acid ratio as is possible.

HOW DO YOU DIGEST A PROTEIN?

Proteins are too large to be absorbed by the

intestines, so they must be broken down before they reach that part of the digestive tract. Physical breakdown of protein begins in the mouth as you chew your food. Chewing food signals your stomach to begin enzymatic secretion of hydrochloric acid and pepsin. This begins the direct process of breaking peptide bonds, which hold proteins together.

From here, smaller protein fractions enter the small intestine. The pancreas releases a series of enzymes, such as cholecystokinin and secretin, which further break down peptide bonds. These small peptides, called oligopeptides, enter the epithelial cells of the small intestine. Another enzyme, aminopeptidase, repeatedly breaks off the N-terminal residue, which is the amino or nitrogen group, from the oligopeptide to make free amino acids.

Free amino acids are absorbed by the intestinal cells and are hydrolyzed to other amino acids before they enter the blood. From here, amino acids are either metabolized by the liver or sent into general circulation to be utilized.

A large proportion of amino acids are absorbed and utilized immediately by the epithelial cells of the small intestine. Intestinal cells are metabolically very active and require a continual supply of the amino acids glutamine and arginine.

WHAT ENERGY FORM
DOES THE BODY PREFER?

The body first uses all of the carbohydrates and fats in the body for energy. Both the brain and heart, two of our most important organs, prefer this form of energy to any other. When fats and carbohydrate sources are low, the body begins to burn dietary protein. If the diet is deficient in dietary energy sources, we begin to break down our own tissue proteins to meet our needs.

CAN YOU BE DEFICIENT IN PROTEIN?

Protein deficiency is also known as protein energy malnutrition (PEM). PEM is found primarily in young children living below poverty level and in third world countries. The World Health Organization estimates that 300 million children worldwide suffer from growth retardation as a result of protein energy malnutrition. Individuals suffering from this condition generally feel fatigue and suffer from increased infections. Death rates in these populations are generally higher as it is more difficult to combat infection with a weakened immune system.

Kwashiorkor is a disease that was first described by pediatrician Cicely Williams, who observed native children in Ghana in 1933. Kwashiorkor literally means "the disease of the deposed baby when the next one is born." This condition commonly affects first-born children who are weaned when a sibling is born. They are forced to eat vegetables that are starchy, with limited protein. They develop severe edema and an enlarged, fatty liver. Ultimately, these children end up with deceptively large bellies, which is due to edema. Kwashiorkor does not occur in second children since they are often allowed to continue nursing, which provides adequate protein and fat.

CAN YOU EAT TOO MUCH?

Most Americans don't have a deficiency of protein in their diets. In fact, the average American consumes 101 grams of protein a day! That is more than double what the average person requires. It has also been estimated that if an individual eats three meals a day from fast-food restaurants, their estimated calorie intake is 5,500 calories, almost double their body's need!

There is a definite concern that individuals in developed countries are overconsuming protein. There is no question that chronic and degenera-

tive diseases are increasing in developed countries at alarming rates. Diseases such as cancer,
diabetes, heart disease, and arthritis have all been
correlated to diets with overconsumption of calories and hydrogenated fats and trans fatty acids.
Because many of the foods high in saturated fat
are from animal-protein sources, it has been suggested that excessive protein consumption may
lead to chronic disease.

CHAPTER 2

WHAT ARE PROTEINS MADE OF?

Proteins are complex molecules, each comprised of its own combination of twenty different amino acids. Proteins each have their own amino acid sequence, or pattern, which is a three-dimensional structure made up of chains, branched molecules, and spheres. The amino acid sequence gives a protein its unique functioning capability, making one protein greatly different from the next.

PRIMARY STRUCTURE

The base sequence of amino acids in a protein is called the primary structure. Understanding a protein's primary structure has led to the detection of many different diseases, specifically genetic diseases. This knowledge has led to early diagnosis and treatment that has helped millions of people.

Amino acids are joined covalently by peptide bonds, which are amide linkages between a carboxyl group of one amino acid and an amino group of another. When two amino acids join together, a protein is formed. When many amino acids are joined together, they form what is called a polypeptide, resulting in a larger protein structure.

Covalent Bond

The sharing of electrons between two atoms, which results in the bonding of the atoms or molecule.

SECONDARY, TERTIARY, AND QUATERNARY STRUCTURES

The larger the protein, the more complex it be-

Alzheimer's Disease

A chronic progressive disorder that accounts for more than 50 percent of all dementia. The disease begins with memory loss and later develops to delusions and paranoia.

comes. A secondary structure is a polypeptide that has formed an arrangement of amino acids that are located next to one another in a linear fashion. The α-helix, β-sheet, and β-bend are examples frequently encountered in secondary proteins. Amyloid protein is a type of β-sheet that is deposited in the brain of individuals suffering from Alzheimer's disease.

The sequence of amino acids or primary structure of a polypeptide will determine its tertiary structure. "Tertiary" refers to the folding of the domains and their final arrangement. "Domains" are the fundamental functional, three-dimensional structural unit of a polypeptide. These polypeptide structures are wound together in a globular form and held in place by strong hydrogen bonds. Immunoglobulins are examples of tertiary proteins.

Immunoglobulins

Proteins that function to assist the immune system in the transport of antibodies against harmful microorganisms such as bacteria and viruses.

Many proteins consist of a single polypeptide chain. Those that consist of two or more subunit polypeptide chains, which may be structurally identical or completely different, are said to have quaternary structure. The subunits may function together or independent of one another. Hemoglobin is an example of a quaternary structure that works cooperatively; oxygen binds to one subunit, increasing the affinity of other subunits for oxygen.

Hemoglobin

The iron-containing pigment of a red blood cell, which carries oxygen from the lungs to tissues.

HOW DOES THE BODY METABOLIZE PROTEIN?

The liver is the primary site in the body where proteins are regulated and metabolized. Every day, all day, proteins are made and broken down. Approximately 60 to 70 percent of amino acids in the body are recycled from old tissue proteins. When a protein is metabolized and broken down, the byproducts that are left behind are utilized to manufacture new amino acids.

Metabolism
The sum of all physical and chemical changes that take place within an organism; all material and energy transformations that occur within living cells.

The breakdown of amino acids in our bodies is a process called catabolism. This, too, occurs in the liver. The first step in catabolism involves the removal of the α-amino group. Once removed, the nitrogen molecule can be incorporated into other compounds or removed from the body.

THE BODY'S ROLE IN MAKING PROTEINS

Recycled amino acids are called endogenous amino acids, or "nonessential" amino acids. They are called nonessential because the body has the ability to self-produce these amino acids, making it not essential to get them in the diet. During the breakdown of amino acids, the α-amino acid is transferred to α-ketoglutarate. This process, called *transamination*, results in the production of an α-keto acid.

Alpha-keto acid is derived from the original amino acid and glutamate. Alpha-ketoglutarate is unique in that it accepts amino groups from other amino acids to allow it to become glutamate. Glutamate produced by transamination can be oxidatively deaminated, that is, the amino group can be removed, or it can be used as an amino group donor in the synthesis of other nonessential amino acids.

The enzyme aminotransferase is the enzyme responsible for transferring amino groups from one carbon skeleton to another. All amino acids, with the exception of lysine and threonine, participate in transamination. There are ten nonessential amino acids that can be metabolized in the body.

Nonessential Amino Acids

- Alanine
- Asparagine
- Aspartate
- Cysteine
- Glutamate
- Glutamine
- Glycine
- Proline
- Serine
- Tyrosine

DEAMINATION: REMOVAL OF WASTE

In contrast to transamination reactions that transfer amino groups, oxidative deamination results in the liberation of amino groups. This reaction occurs mostly in the liver but also happens to some degree in the kidney. After being processed in the liver, the amino group becomes ammonia and, ultimately, urea. Urea is the largest disposal form of amino groups derived from amino acids. It accounts for 90 percent of the nitrogen-containing components of urine.

WHAT ABOUT THE REST OF THE AMINO ACIDS?

Essential amino acids are those that the body can't synthesize on its own. The only way to obtain essential amino acids is through the diet. There are eight essential amino acids. When essential amino acids are present in the diet, the body can make an adequate supply of nonessential amino acids. If one essential amino acid is low, even in the presence of a high-protein diet, the body will be unable to synthesize all the necessary nonessentials.

Essential Amino Acids

- Isoleucine
- Phenylalanine
- Leucine
- Threonine
- Lysine
- Tryptophan
- Methionine
- Valine

Two amino acids are considered semi-essential. They can be made in the body to a certain extent; however, they become essential for some individuals when the body's demand increases. They are essential for all children and during times of increased growth, such as during pregnancy, lactation, and puberty.

Semi-Essential Amino Acids

- Arginine
- Histidine

While not considered essential building blocks of human protein tissue, many other amino acids that exist in nature do participate in many important metabolic functions. Some of these amino acids are very similar to, or are derived from other amino acids. Chapter 5 discusses several of the therapeutic uses of these amino acids.

Amino Acids Not Found in Body Proteins*

- Carnitine
- Ornithine
- Taurine

but are important for metabolic function

THE IMPORTANCE OF COFACTORS

Our bodies can become deficient in nonessential amino acids when our diet is lacking in protein in general, or a particular vitamin and mineral. For example, vitamin B_6 in its active form, pyridoxal-5-phosphate, is a cofactor necessary to generate protein synthesis in the liver. When this vitamin is absent, or depleted in the body, nonessential amino acids are not made efficiently.

Some protein enzymes require a non-protein cofactor for a biochemical reaction to occur in the body. As mentioned above, when a cofactor is deficient, enzymatic activity is limited and therefore reactions are slowed down in the body. If this deficiency persists over a long period of time, there is a shift in metabolism and the body begins to manifest a disease process.

CHAPTER 3

ROLE OF PROTEINS IN THE BODY

Proteins are needed to initiate every biochemical process in the body, as well as provide us with an invaluable source of energy. Without proteins, the body would simply shut down. By understanding the wide range of jobs proteins perform, you can begin to understand your body's need for complete proteins.

ARE THERE DIFFERENT TYPES OF PROTEINS?

As discussed in Chapter 2, there are different sizes of polypeptides, or proteins. Proteins can be divided into two categories, structural and globular. When you think of a structural protein, think of animal hide or leather, or your own hair. A structural protein is solid matter composed of long, thin filaments. A good example of filaments working together as a unit is muscle contraction, which occurs when two protein filaments glide across each other.

A globular protein is entirely different in composition. It is a combination of a few molecules in a globular shape, rather than a long, thin strand. The most important example of a globular protein is an enzyme. Having this globular structure allows enzymes to be soluble in a solution, or liquid form. Digestive enzymes work-

Enzyme
A substance that comes in contact with another substance inside of a cell and causes a chemical reaction to occur, but which remains unchanged in the process.

ing to help us absorb and process our food exemplifies one enzyme system in the body.

By understanding the different types of proteins, you will be better able to understand their functions. In the remainder of this chapter, we will explore their diverse functions.

ROLE OF ENZYMES

As mentioned previously, proteins are responsible for nearly every chemical reaction that occurs in the body. These reactions are mediated by enzymes, which are protein catalysts that increase the rate of reaction without themselves being changed in the process. The amount of enzymes available in the body determines the rate at which a chemical event can occur. Therefore, if an enzyme is deficient, there will be a slower reaction.

Among the many chemical reactions that can occur, enzymes selectively channel a substrate, or reactant, into the proper pathway. Ultimately, enzymes direct every metabolic pathway in the body.

Enzymes also rely on cofactors. Cofactors often come in the form of a vitamin or nutrient. Again, if a particular vitamin or nutrient is deficient, enzymes won't be able to cause an efficient chemical reaction, resulting in a limited amount of amino acid.

Several thousand enzymes have been discovered to date and virtually every one is a protein!

TRANSPORTATION AND STORAGE

Proteins are required to carry different molecules throughout the body. Proteins have a unique ability to transport substances across cell membranes that other molecules can't penetrate.

Hemoglobin is a type of protein that is responsible for carrying oxygen in a red blood cell. Myoglobin, which is a similar protein, is responsible for carrying oxygen in muscle tissue. Ferritin is a protein that assists in the storage of iron, and ultimately stores blood in the liver.

Without proteins for transportation and storage, we would not have blood to nourish our bodies!

CELL AND TISSUE GROWTH

Our bodies need a constant supply of amino acids to build the proteins that create tissue. Throughout our daily lives, we constantly manufacture new tissues, such as hair, teeth, skin, and nails. Other tissue becomes worn out, such as the tissue in our joints, and needs constant replacement.

Red blood cells and skin cells last about a month, while the cells that line our digestive system only last two weeks. When these cells die and slough off, our bodies need new healthy tissue to replace them.

Slough
A shedding process the body undergoes to replace old dead tissue with new healthy tissue.

When healing from trauma or surgery, our bodies require more protein production to help our tissue regenerate quickly. It is only through the regeneration of new tissue that we can become healthy again!

MECHANICAL SUPPORT

Collagen, the most abundant protein found in the human body, is a type of structural protein that is fibrous in nature. Collagen is responsible for giving strength and support to tissues such as skin and bone that undergo continual wear and tear.

Although collagen is found throughout the body, its type and organization is dictated by the particular structural role it is required to perform. In some tissues, collagen may be bundled in tight parallel fibers to provide great strength, such as in a tendon. In the cornea of the eye, collagen is stacked in such a way that light can be transmitted with a limited amount of scattering. Collagen in the bone occurs as fibers that are arranged at an angle to one another; this way, they can resist mechanical shear from any direction.

Athletes that work out two or more hours a day rely on the body's ability to manufacture new collagen, which keeps their joints healthy and strong and prevents injury. The amino acid sequence of collagen is unique in that glycine, the smallest amino acid, is found in every third position along the peptide chain. Clearly, the importance of this amino acid in our diet is indisputable.

COORDINATION AND MOTION

Proteins are a major component of muscle contraction. Muscle contraction occurs when two fibrous protein filaments glide across each other. On a smaller scale, sperm are propelled in motion by their flagella, which are composed of contractile units made of proteins. Without proteins, we could not create life!

ELASTICITY

In contrast to collagen, which forms tensile and tough fibers, elastin is a connective tissue protein with elasticlike properties. Elastin fibers can be stretched to several times their normal length; they then recoil back to their original shape when the stretching force is relaxed. Elastin is found in the lungs, for example, where a stretch recoil mechanism allows each breath. Elastin is also found in blood vessels, creating a pumping effect, and in ligaments that support our joints.

Antigen
A type of protein that the body recognizes as foreign, such as a bacteria, virus, fungi, pollen, or yeast.

IMMUNE PROTECTION

Antibodies are highly specific proteins that are responsible for detecting a foreign substance, or antigen, when it enters the body. The body will produce a specific antibody to respond to an antigen and inactivate it. Different invaders require specific antibody proteins, thus the body is under constant surveillance to protect itself from getting overwhelmed and ultimately sick.

NERVE GENERATION AND IMPULSES

Our nervous system is responsible for keeping the body in balance. When a specific stimulus triggers the nervous system, it responds with an appropriate reaction. This can't occur without a receptor site awaiting the stimulus. These receptor sites are made of protein complexes and are responsible for transmitting nerve messages from cell to cell.

Receptor
A cell component that combines with a drug, hormone, or chemical mediator to alter the function of a cell with a physiological response.

FLUID BALANCE

Proteins have the unique ability to regulate the amount of fluid within a cell. The amount of protein within a cell will determine the cell's water content, as water is attracted to protein. When protein levels are low, fluid imbalances result. This type of system is important to prevent dehydration, as well as to enhance muscle and nerve cell function.

ENZYMES AS A DIAGNOSTIC TOOL

In addition to stimulating metabolic pathways in our bodies, enzymes can help diagnose disease.

Plasma enzymes are found in the blood and are classified into two major groups. The first is a small group of enzymes; these are actively secreted into plasma by select organs. The second is a larger group of enzymes that are released from the cell in normal cell turnover. These enzymes are intracellular and have no physiological function in our bodies.

Plasma
The fluid, noncellular part of blood. When you have your blood drawn, it is spun at a high rate and the serum part of plasma is analyzed.

In a healthy individual, levels of plasma enzymes are constant and represent the rate at which the cell releases into the plasma and the rate at which it is removed from the plasma and excreted. The presence of elevated enzyme activity is typically indicative of tissue damage that is accompanied by an increase in the rate of cell turnover.

The liver and the heart are two major organs in which enzyme levels are checked to assess tissue damage. Oftentimes with routine blood work, liver enzymes are checked. Alanine aminotransferase (ALT) is one example of a liver enzyme. When this enzyme is elevated, it suggests the possibility of liver tissue damage. This enzymatic test is nonspecific and requires further diagnostic workup before conclusions can be drawn.

Heart enzymes such as creatine kinase (CK) and lactate dehydrogenase (LDH) are more specific and, therefore, can be used to make a diagnosis. When these enzymes are elevated, it typically indicates that an individual has had a myocardial infarction, or heart attack. When a patient comes to the emergency room with chest pain, these two enzymes are measured right away.

CHAPTER 4

BENEFITS OF PROTEIN SUPPLEMENTATION

For many individuals, therapeutic protein supplementation can be of benefit. For some, a protein shake or smoothie is a great way to start the day. In this chapter, you will learn about various protein supplements and how they can benefit your health.

Protein supplementation comes in all shapes, sizes, and flavors. You can buy a protein supplement as a complete protein such as whey, soy, or rice powder, or you can buy individual amino acids. This chapter focuses on the differences between complete protein supplements and how they can suit your individual needs.

As mentioned earlier, complete proteins, meaning proteins that contain all twenty amino acids, are found primarily in animal products. As a consumer, your choices for nonfood protein supplementation are whey, soy, or rice supplements. Of these, only whey comes from an animal source and is a stand-alone complete protein. Soy and rice protein supplements can be made complete with the addition of specific amino acids to the finished product.

WHEY PROTEIN

Whey is a protein complex that is derived from cow's milk. Milk contains two primary sources of protein, casein and whey. Little Miss Muffet, who ate her curds and whey, drank her whey, as it is the liquid part of milk. During the processing of protein powder, whey becomes a solid, or powder.

Why Whey?

Whey is a complete protein, containing all twenty amino acids. Additionally, whey contains essential amino acids in higher concentrations than in other vegetable sources such as soy, corn, and wheat gluten. In addition to having a full spectrum of amino acids, the amino acids found in whey are efficiently absorbed and utilized relative to individual amino acid supplements.

Cysteine is one of the most important amino acids naturally found in high concentration in whey protein. Cysteine is helpful in eradicating toxins and is a precursor to the body's most potent antioxidant, glutathione. Whey is also an excellent source of branched-chained amino acids. These are essential for tissue growth and repair.

Human milk, or breast milk, is the most important building block for infants. It sets the foundation for development of the nervous and immune systems, and provides superior nutrition for increased cellular growth demands. In Appendix B, there is a chart comparing the amino acid profile of milk from both humans and cows. As you will see, the amino acid profile of whey is comparable to that of human milk, making it a highly beneficial source to continue getting the nutrition we need.

Immune-Enhancing Effects

Whey proteins contain a wide range of protein complexes that exhibit immune-enhancing properties. These complexes include lactoferrin, immunoglobulins, beta-lactoglobulin, and alpha-lactalbumin.

Lactoferrin is an iron-binding protein found in all forms of milk, including human and cow. It provides iron to the body and is an important immune modulator. Lactoferrin is responsible for stimulating the immune system to respond to infections, tumors, and cancers.

Other immune cells known as immunoglobulins are also present in whey. They function to transport antibodies that are necessary to fight viruses, bacteria, and other foreign invaders. They form the "first line of defense" against organisms entering the digestive system.

Immunoglobulins are transferred from a mother to her fetus in utero, and also through breast milk. Children develop their immune systems by ingesting antibodies present in the milk. The immunoglobulins in whey are comparable; they are so potent that they are able to eradicate bacteria such as *E. coli, Salmonella,* and *Shigella,* and yeast such as *Candida albicans,*

Beta-lactoglobulin and alpha-lactalbumin comprise the majority of proteins found in milk. Alpha-lactalbumin has a wide variety of amino acids, including a readily available source of essential and branched-chain amino acids.

Are There Other Health Benefits from Whey?

Besides its potent immune activity, studies have shown whey to be effective in the treatment of heart disease, osteoporosis, and cancer. The rationale for this is in part due to the ability of the body to convert whey protein into glutathione. A fair amount of research has been done suggesting that whey improves muscle strength and body composition, especially when combined with exercise.

Glutathione

An important antioxidant that is made up of glycine, glutamate, and cysteine. It works to prevent tissue damage.

Glutathione, which is made in the body, is important for the safe metabolism of free radicals (molecules with an unpaired electron), helping to prevent disease. It protects against radiation and oxidative damage that can permanently damage tissues in the body.

Many theories of aging are based upon the

theory of free-radical formation. A reduction of glutathione in the body results in increased free-radical formation, and ultimately chronic disease. Free radicals that stay within cells cause cellular damage, DNA damage, and may even cause cell death or tumor formation.

Is Whey for Everyone?

Casein
The solid portion of milk, or curd.

Because some individuals have sensitivity to dairy products, whey may not be suitable for everyone. Most people, however, have an inability to digest casein protein. Casein protein is completely removed during the processing of whey, making it more tolerable and less allergenic. Additionally, lactose is found in negligible amounts.

SOY PROTEIN

For years, vegetarians and vegans have been consuming soy as an alternative to meat, poultry, and other animal-based products. In recent years, soy consumption has risen as health food stores have begun to carry a huge variety of soy products, from soy energy bars to soy protein shakes.

The Benefits of Soy

To date, several dozen clinical trials have been conducted on humans, demonstrating a favorable health effect of diets containing soy. Most recently, the U.S. Food and Drug Administration (FDA) has allowed soy manufacturers to claim on their food label that a diet containing 25 grams of soy protein daily may reduce the risk of heart disease.

Soy is most notably used by women going through menopause. Many women notice a reduction in menopausal symptoms, such as hot flashes and mental function, when they consume soy. This is because soy is high in isoflavones, such as genistein and daidzein, which are in a larger family of phytoestrogens. (Phytoestrogens have the ability to bind to estrogen receptors in the body and can have a mild estrogenic effect in specific female tissues, ultimately reducing menopausal complaints.)

Phytoestrogens are found in most plants to some degree, but in plants such as soy, it is found in large concentrations. Phytoestrogens have a unique ability to bind weakly to estrogen receptors in the body, creating either a weak estrogenic effect or a mild antiestrogenic effect. This type of selective binding can be beneficial in a variety of health conditions that effect women, such as heart disease, fibrocystic breast disease, and osteoporosis.

Phytoestrogens
Plant-derived substances that are able to activate estrogen receptors in animals, including humans.

Is Soy a Complete Protein?

Some levels of essential amino acids in soy are not as high as those found in animal products. Many soy enthusiasts would argue that soy does contain the full spectrum of amino acids. However, thorough analysis has revealed something entirely different. It has been discovered that soy protein lacks the essential amino acid methionine.

Is Soy for Everyone?

Soy is definitely not for everyone. A good amount of research has been done suggesting that individuals with estrogen-sensitive cancers, such as breast, prostate, ovarian, or uterine cancer, should not use soy products. This is partly because phytoestrogens occupy estrogen-receptor sights in the body, thereby stimulating estrogen in some while decreasing it in others. It is safest to avoid soy if you have thyroid disease or breast or uterine cancer.

Soy also has higher levels of phytic acid, which may disrupt how the body utilizes certain minerals such as calcium, magnesium, copper, iron, and zinc.

Soy appears to inhibit thyroid hormone production in some individuals. In addition, soy can interfere with thyroid hormone medication. Soy supplements or soy foods should be taken several hours before or after thyroid hormone medication. Recent studies also suggest that soy formula for infants may perpetuate thyroid disease later in life.

RICE PROTEIN

Rice protein supplements are an excellent choice when looking for a vegan, hypoallergenic protein. Whey, which is derived from animal proteins, is not an option for some vegetarians or vegans. Soy protein is often difficult to digest and can cause stomach upset. According to the net protein utilization (NPU) system, rice protein is better assimilated by the body when compared to soy.

Rice protein has a mild, creamy flavor and is well suited for the individual with food allergies. For those forced to use feeding tubes, such as the elderly or the severely ill, rice protein can be used for tube feeding.

Is Rice for Everyone?

Very few people have an allergic response, or sensitivity, to rice. Both whey and soy proteins exhibit a broader range of amino acids; however, in a highly sensitive individual who can't tolerate whey or soy, rice is an excellent option. To obtain all amino acids, a complete diet must accompany rice protein supplementation.

Some individual dietary needs require an increase in carbohydrates, especially if weight gain is a concern. Rice protein typically has a higher carbohydrate count compared to whey or soy protein. For some athletes who require extra carbohydrates for energy utilization, rice protein may be of benefit.

HOW MUCH PROTEIN DO WE NEED ANYWAY?

Protein should account for at least 15 to 20 percent of the calories in a balanced diet. A normal adult requires approximately 0.36 grams of protein per pound of body weight. That means if you weigh 140 pounds, you will need 50 grams of protein a day. This is equivalent to 2 ounces of pure protein. Healthy adults require approximately 45–65 grams of protein a day.

Does Anyone Truly Need Higher Amounts of Protein?

Many athletes, because of the increased demand on their bodies, do require slightly more protein. Protein is needed to repair tissue that constantly undergoes wear and tear with endurance, extreme, and elite-level sports.

Pregnant women also need to increase their protein intake to between 90 and 100 grams of protein a day. During the nine months of gestation, the fetus undergoes a tremendous amount of growth and puts increased energy demands on mom. It is also important to keep protein intake up during lactation.

Should Anyone Limit His or Her Protein Intake Intentionally?

Individuals with chronic kidney disease should limit their protein intake. The kidney is the primary means for excreting byproducts when amino acids are made in the body. Therefore:

more protein = more byproducts =
more work for the kidneys!

CHAPTER 5

WHEN TO USE INDIVIDUAL AMINO ACIDS

Amino acid supplementation can be extremely beneficial in a wide variety of medical conditions. Because proteins play so many roles in the body, virtually every amino acid can impact health positively. However, not all amino acids are used therapeutically. Those that are most commonly used are discussed in this chapter.

As with other nutritional supplements, amino acid supplementation should not be continued indefinitely. To prevent an imbalance of other amino acids, either discontinue use of individual amino acids after six months or supplement with a basic amino acid mixture or protein powder supplement that offers a complete amino acid profile.

THE ESSENTIAL AMINO ACIDS

Because essential amino acids can't be manufactured in our bodies, we need to eat a balanced diet. Some individuals, for one reason or another, are not able to consume adequate protein to achieve physiologic let alone therapeutic levels of a particular amino acid. As you will see in this chapter, and in Appendix A at the back of the book, amino acids, when used therapeutically, are often prescribed at very high dosages.

Lysine

Lysine is an essential amino acid that interacts to a large degree both in the formation and in the utilization of other amino acids. The most prominent functions of lysine include synthesizing connective tissue, brain neurotransmission, and carbohydrate metabolism. During metabolism, lysine is degraded to acetyl CoA, a critical component of the body's energy cycle.

Lysine appears to help the body absorb and conserve calcium, as well as decrease the body's rate of calcium excretion. Because of this, studies have found lysine to have a role in the prevention of osteoporosis.

Lysine has the ability to interfere with the replication of the herpes virus, and can be used preventively and therapeutically for individuals with the herpes virus. Lysine has also been used in clinical trials in the treatment of cold sores.

Lysine is an antagonist of the amino acid arginine. Arginine levels can therefore become deficient if lysine is taken in high amounts for an extended period of time. Animal studies have also revealed that if high amounts of lysine are taken, individuals may be at risk of developing gallstones.

Methionine

Methionine is a sulfur-containing amino acid that is essential for normal metabolism and growth. In the body, methionine is converted to S-adenosyl methionine (SAMe), which is considered the active form of methionine.

SAMe is an important biological methylating agent. Methylation by SAMe is critical for the stabilization of many proteins, including myelin. In the methylation cycle, SAMe releases a methyl (CH3) group from its structure to ultimately form homocysteine. If there is deficient methionine or nutrient cofactors, then there are resultant defects in homocysteine metabolism. Such defects can lead to cognitive decline, dementia, or cardiovascular disease.

As a methyl donor, SAMe is also involved in

RNA and DNA
Nucleic acids found in every living thing. They are responsible for providing unique differentiation between species.

the breakdown of estrogen, melatonin synthesis, and histamine degradation. It is required for RNA and DNA synthesis and the metabolism of vitamins and fats. It has the ability to increase the body's level of glutathione, making it especially important for liver detoxification.

SAMe also appears to have significant analgesic effects, suggesting its use in the treatment of osteoarthritis. Additionally, SAMe plays a significant role in maintaining cartilage health in our joints. In a number of clinical trials, SAMe at a dose of 400 mg three times a day has demonstrated its effects to be more significant than many standard medications such as nonsteroidal anti-inflammatory drugs (NSAIDs). In addition, SAMe appears to have fewer side effects.

SAMe has been effectively studied in the treatment of depression in several clinical trials. At a dose of 400 mg four times a day, SAMe proved more favorable than MAO inhibitors and tricyclic antidepressants, drugs traditionally used to treat depression. Methionine is readily absorbed across the blood-brain barrier and is converted into epinephrine and norepinephrine. It has the potential to be especially useful for treating postpartum depression and depression associated with drug and alcohol withdrawal.

Dementia
A broad term used to describe a decrease in cognitive ability, including memory loss.

Individuals with AIDS tend to have lower levels of methionine. It has been suggested that AIDS may cause broad-spectrum amino acid deficiencies because of the disease's muscle-wasting tendencies. Taking high doses of methionine has demonstrated a positive effect on people with AIDS-related dementia.

It should be noted that diets high in methionine and low in B vitamins place individuals at increased risk of elevated homocysteine levels. An elevated homocysteine level may increase your risk of heart disease. This can be remedied by making sure that you have adequate levels of all B vitamins, including folic acid.

Tryptophan: 5-HTP

Tryptophan is the essential amino acid that is least abundant in food. It is responsible for the production of the neurotransmitter serotonin. Deficiency of serotonin has significant clinical implications for depression and insomnia. Tryptophan has demonstrated an ability to ease these conditions, as well as improve symptoms of impaired memory, concentration, and evaluative judgment.

In 1989, the Centers for Disease Control reported a link between tryptophan supplementation and a condition called eosinophilia-myalgia syndrome. The FDA recalled all products that contained tryptophan, except for infant formulas and parenteral formulas. It was subsequently found that a manufacturer in Japan was using a new bacterial strain to synthesize tryptophan in their laboratory. It was this strain that was producing the toxic byproducts responsible for eosinophilia-myalgia syndrome.

A metabolite of tryptophan, 5-hydroxy tryptophan (5-HTP), has proven to be more effective in treating similar conditions. 5-HTP is an intermediary metabolite in the pathway between tryptophan and serotonin. Some individuals with depression have difficulty converting 5-HTP naturally in their bodies, and clinical trials have shown that supplementation with 5-HTP can be just as effective as traditional antidepressants.

In a double-blind study conducted on patients with fibromyalgia, after thirty days of supplementation with 5-HTP, there appeared to be a significant decline in tender points. Patients also had less morning pain and stiffness, better sleep patterns, and less fatigue. Often individuals with a diagnosis of fibromyalgia have symptoms that include insomnia and depression.

Enhanced therapeutic benefits can be obtained when supplementation with both tryptophan and its metabolite 5-HTP is used in combination with vitamin B_6 and niacinamide. These nutrients, in combination, create a synergistic effect to increase neurotransmitter metabolism.

Phenylalanine

Phenylalanine, in the "L" configuration, can be converted in the body to tyrosine and subsequently L-dopa, norepinephrine, and epinephrine. These important neurotransmitters play a significant role in moderating brain chemistry. As a result, phenylalanine, or more specifically DL-phenylalanine, has been used successfully to treat depression.

DL-phenylalanine has shown moderate success in treating individuals with chronic pain by inhibiting endorphins and enkephalins in the body. Endorphins and enkephalins have mood-enhancing and analgesic effects.

DL-phenylalanine has successfully decreased symptoms of rigidity and depression in individuals with Parkinson's disease. Unfortunately, it does not appear to help with tremors associated with this condition.

Phenylalanine may be more commonly associated with the disease phenlyketonuria (PKU). PKU was first discovered in 1934 when it was realized that 1 percent of the institutionalized mentally retarded population had high levels of phenylpyruvic acid. Ultimately, it was determined that this genetic condition occurs in 1 in 5,000 live births, accounting for 1 percent of the population. In those with PKU, the body does not convert phenylalanine into tyrosine. Fortunately, today it can be detected and treated promptly, preventing many children from becoming severely retarded.

The Branched-Chain Amino Acids: Leucine, Isoleucine, and Valine

Among the essential amino acids are the branched-chain amino acids: leucine, isoleucine, and valine. They have been coined "branched-chain" because of their unique biochemical makeup. They are responsible for maintaining muscle tissue by preventing muscle breakdown during exercise. They are unique in that they are metabolized primarily by peripheral tissue rather than in the liver.

Therapeutically, they are of benefit because they bypass the liver for metabolism and are more readily available for the body. Intravenous administration of branched-chain amino acids (BCAAs) on their own, or in combination with other amino acids, is thought to be of benefit when there is physiological stress on the body. Skeletal and heart muscle can use these amino acids for energy.

BCAAs are most commonly used in the athletic arena. When used in moderation, BCAAs may allow athletes to recover quickly after a workout. Studies reveal mixed reports suggesting that BCAAs do not generally improve exercise performance; however, in extreme conditions, they can prolong endurance.

Smaller studies have revealed that BCAAs may be beneficial for individuals with kidney failure. When undergoing dialysis, patients treated with BCAAs had improved breathing and quality of sleep.

In the treatment of children with PKU, regular use of branched-chain amino acids resulted in improved test scores as well as an increase in mental functioning.

THE NONESSENTIAL AMINO ACIDS

As mentioned in Chapter 2, nonessential amino acids are those that the body can make on its own and are found in body proteins. Deficient levels of nonessential amino acids may be found when insufficient or non-bioavailable protein is consumed.

Cysteine: N-Acetyl Cysteine

Cysteine, a versatile sulfur-containing amino acid, is most commonly used as the derivative N-acetyl cysteine. Because of its sulfur component, cysteine has unique binding and structural capabilities in the body. Cysteine is used by the body to produce the amino acid taurine, and is a component of the antioxidant glutathione.

Cysteine has many important functions in the body. It can serve as a source of energy by converting to glucose when the body is depleted of carbohydrate stores. Cysteine strengthens the protective lining of the stomach and intestines, which may help to prevent damage from aspirin and other similar drugs. It also may play an important role in the communication of lymphocytes, important immune-modulating cells.

N-acetyl cysteine (NAC) is becoming the most widely used therapeutic source of cysteine, as it is the most easily absorbed form. NAC has the ability to thin mucus, allowing it to flow more freely. This is extremely beneficial in conditions such as sinusitis, bronchitis, pneumonia, cystic fibrosis, and asthma. It can be taken acutely in higher doses such as 500 mg for up to five days, or long-term at 200 mg twice a day.

Blood levels of cysteine and glutathione are low in individuals with HIV. Studies suggest that NAC is capable of improving T-cell counts in HIV-infected individuals and preventing HIV from progressing to AIDS.

Historically, the most widely accepted use of

NAC is as an antidote to acetaminophen (Tylenol) and heavy metal poisoning. NAC, when administered intravenously or orally within twenty-four hours, has the ability to restore glutathione levels in the liver to prevent liver toxicity. It is most effective if given within eight hours.

It is suspected that NAC has the ability to pull heavy metals across tissues, which are then combined with glutathione and excreted in the bowel. There are no published clinical trials demonstrating this effect, so it should only be considered under proper medical supervision.

Therapeutic benefit with NAC supplementation has also been demonstrated in conditions such as heart disease, hepatitis, and Sjögren's syndrome, as well as in the prevention and treatment of some cancers.

Glutamine

Glutamine is the most abundant amino acid in the body. It is found predominantly in our bones, muscles, and blood. It is considered to be conditionally essential, meaning it only needs to be supplemented during times of stress, as in the case of acute bowel inflammation. It is made naturally in the body, formed from glutamic acid. When the body is stressed, it utilizes glutamine from muscle tissue, making the body's demand greater than what it can synthesize.

Conditionally Essential Amino Acid

An amino acid that can be considered essential during times of physiologic stress, including severe inflammation or burns.

Glutamine is the preferred energy source for enterocytes, the cells that line the digestive system, and is involved in more metabolic processes than any other amino acid. It is converted to glucose when more glucose is required by the body for energy. And it helps sustain the body's immune system. Immune cells that rapidly divide, such as lymphocytes and macrophages, rely on glutamine. Athletes who overtrain can become depleted in glutamine, making them more susceptible to infection.

In the intestines, glutamine replacement is essential to repair tissue damaged by inflammation. In individuals with inflammatory bowel disease, such as Crohn's disease and ulcerative colitis, supplementing with glutamine is important to help maintain weight and intestinal tissue integrity. It has also proven beneficial in repairing intestinal tissue lining in individuals with peptic ulcer disease.

In a study published in the journal *Nutrition*, critically ill people were found to be more likely to survive if they were given intravenous glutamine supplementation. The digestive systems of critically ill patients tend to have increased permeability, decreasing nutrient absorption. Glutamine appears to improve the immune system and increase wound healing in these individuals.

In individuals with HIV/AIDS, there appears to be glutamine deficiency resulting in muscle protein wasting. Approximately 20 percent of individuals with AIDS also have severe intestinal permeability. A double-blind, placebo-controlled study was conducted on sixty-eight HIV-infected patients with documented weight loss. They were given 14 grams of glutamine per day. The glutamine supplemented group gained lean body mass and total body weight, while the placebo group lost lean body mass. There also appeared to be an increase in CD4 and CD8 cells for the glutamine-treated group, demonstrating a positive immune response for eight weeks. At eight weeks the group given glutamine gained 3 kg of lean response, as well.

The use of glutamine in individuals with cancer remains controversial. In laboratory studies, glutamine added to tumor cells increased cellular, or tumor, growth. However, in human studies, glutamine supplementation did not appear to increase tumor growth. In fact, in one animal study, glutamine supplementation reduced tumor growth by 40 percent and stimulated natural killer cell activity.

Natural Killer Cells

Cells that are often the first immune responders to a viral infection. They also have important anti-cancer activity and enhance inflammatory response in bacterial infection.

Many forms of chemotherapy cause diarrhea as a side effect. Glutamine supplementation, when given simultaneously with chemotherapy, can reduce diarrhea and other digestive complaints. Doses of glutamine used in cancer therapeutics are very high and should only be considered under supervision of a health-care professional.

Glycine

Glycine is found in high concentrations in prostate fluid and may play a role in maintaining prostate health. Studies have demonstrated that glycine has a therapeutic use for people with schizophrenia. Greater benefits were noticed when glycine was taken in combination with equal amounts of alanine and glutamic acid.

Glycine has proven to be beneficial in improving memory and cognition by enhancing a chemical receptor site in the brain.

Tyrosine

Tyrosine is a nonessential amino acid formed in the body as an intermediary step in the conversion of phenylalanine to norepinephrine. It is also a precursor to the neurotransmitters epinephrine and dopamine. Vitamin B_6, folic acid, and copper are necessary for the conversion of L-tyrosine into various neurotransmitters. Tyrosine is also an essential nutrient in the formation of thyroid hormone.

Tyrosine has been used in the treatment of narcolepsy but is most commonly used in the treatment of depression. Some forms of depression are due to an insufficient amount of epinephrine and dopamine being available. In other cases, depression results from the body's inability to convert phenylalanine to tyrosine. Taking tyrosine can therefore be beneficial.

Because tyrosine acts as a precursor to neurotransmitters such as L-dopa, it has been explored as a therapeutic treatment for Parkinson's disease. Supplementation with tyrosine can increase cerebrospinal fluid levels of homovanillic acid, a major dopamine metabolite, and increase dopamine turnover. Tyrosine appears to have fewer side effects than L-dopa and should not be used simultaneously.

Tyrosine has also been used therapeutically in individuals with PKU, Alzheimer's disease, and people under a lot of stress. One study conducted on night watchmen in the military found that when supplementing with tyrosine, soldiers were able to stay more alert and focused.

SEMI-ESSENTIAL AMINO ACIDS

Under normal circumstances, the following amino acids are considered nonessential, meaning the body can make an adequate supply. However, during times when the body's growth utilizes its inherent supply, the body's demand requires more supply thorough the diet, thereby qualifying it as semi-essential.

Histidine

Histidine is the precursor to histamine, an immune cell released by the body during inflammation or an allergic reaction. Limited research has shown that individuals with rheumatoid arthritis may have low levels of histidine. It has been suggested that people with rheumatoid disease would benefit from supplementation with histidine.

Arginine

Arginine is a semi-essential amino acid that is responsible for many biochemical and physiological reactions in the body. It can be synthesized in the body from glutamic acid in a series of reactions. Ultimately, arginine is rapidly synthesized into ornithine or broken down to form urea in the urea cycle. Arginine is broken down so quickly that the body has difficulty keeping up its supply. In addition, it is poorly digested.

Arginine's primary role in the body is to feed the urea cycle, which is essential for ammonia detoxification. Over 50 percent of arginine in the body feeds this cycle. The remaining arginine in the body is used in wound healing, to promote hormone secretion, to stimulate immune function, or as a precursor to nitric oxide.

Most recently, arginine received attention for its role as a biological precursor to nitric oxide (NO), an endogenous messenger molecule involved in a variety of physiological effects in the cardiovascular system. It appears to be extremely important in maintaining normal blood pressure, cholesterol, and heart function, in controlling inflammation, and as an antioxidant. Arginine has demonstrated its usefulness in the treatment of angina, congestive heart failure, hypertension, and intermittent claudication.

Nitric oxide metabolism defects also appear to play a role in the development of erectile dysfunction. In clinical trials a dose of 2.8 grams of arginine a day has proven to be effective in improving erectile function.

Arginine supplementation has been studied with positive results in men with infertility. Arginine is required by the body to make healthy, mobile sperm. In a study conducted over fifty years ago, it was found that feeding men an arginine-deficient diet for nine days caused sperm counts to decrease by approximately 90 percent and the amount of nonmotile sperm to increase tenfold!

Interstitial Cystitis
A urinary condition that resembles a chronic urinary tract infection but appears normal in laboratory tests.

Interstitial cystitis is a very difficult condition to treat. Supplementation with arginine in clinical trials has resulted in a significant decrease in symptoms such as pain with urination, pain in the lower abdomen, and urinary frequency.

In individuals with significant burns and trauma, the body's arginine reserves are greatly reduced. Additionally, there is a dramatic increase in arginine oxidation, making what is there unusable. These cases exemplify arginine's function as a conditionally essential amino acid; that is, arginine is "essential" following injury and supplementation becomes important.

Diets that are high in arginine have been known to promote the growth of herpes simplex virus, especially when dietary lysine levels are low. Dietary arginine is found in many animal products, but it is also high in chocolate and nuts, particularly peanuts.

THE SMALL PROTEINS

There are a handful of di- and tripeptides that are very important therapeutically. They are combinations of two to three different amino acids that play critical roles in our bodies. Without them, as you will see, we simply would not survive.

Glutathione

Glutathione is a tripeptide composed of cysteine, glutamine, and glycine. It is an extremely important cell protector, and is found in every living cell in our bodies. Glutathione is most active in the body in its reduced form, simply called reduced glutathione. When supplementing with glutathione, always make sure it is in its reduced form, as the body has difficulty absorbing non-reduced glutathione.

Glutathione is the most important antioxidant found naturally in our bodies. It is an essential part of the body's detoxification system since it binds to fat-soluble toxins and transforms them into water-soluble toxins that are easily excreted. Because of its role as an antioxidant and detoxifier, gluta-thione is important in the prevention of cancer.

Some studies reveal that intravenous glu-tathione, when administered simultaneously with chemotherapy, can reduce the side effects and increase the effectiveness of the chemotherapy.

Many chronic health conditions can be associ-ated with a glutathione deficiency. Ultimately, most chronic diseases can be looked at as a fail-ure in the body's natural ability to break down and eliminate toxins and thereby prevent oxida-tive and tissue damage. When glutathione levels are adequate, this body failure usually does not occur to the point of disease progression. Dis-eases associated with low glutathione levels are diabetes, low sperm counts, liver disease, cataracts, HIV, cancer, and pulmonary fibrosis. Cigarette smokers are also low in glutathione.

Other nutrients that affect glutathione levels are alpha-lipoic acid, glutamine, methionine, and S-adenosyl methionine (SAMe). The body requires vitamins B_6, riboflavin (B_5), and selenium in order to manufacture glutathione. Whey protein is used therapeutically as a means of increasing intracel-lular glutathione levels.

Carnosine

Carnosine is a small protein molecule composed of histidine and alanine. It is found in high concentration in skeletal muscle, heart muscle, and in the brain. Its role in the body is not completely understood, but we do know it is a potent anti-oxidant, protects us against radiation damage, improves cardiac function, and promotes wound healing.

Therapeutically, carnosine in the form of zinc-L-carnosine is protective against peptic ulcer formation and assists in the healing of existing ulcers. It also helps to eradicate *H. pylori,* a bacteria that is known to increase the risk of developing ulcers.

Zinc-L-carnosine may also be effective in treating severe gingivitis that is sometimes caused by chemotherapy. It appears to be more effective when used in combination with sodium alginate.

CHAPTER 6

SHOPPING FOR PROTEIN AND AMINO ACID SUPPLEMENTS

Now that you have begun to understand the importance of protein in your life, the following guidelines will provide you with simple information to assist you in making choices while standing in the supplement aisle at a health food store. At the very least, you will discover that you have choices both in quality and price.

SHOPPING FOR THE RIGHT AMINO ACID SUPPLEMENT

Some nutritional supplement companies have taken amino acid therapeutics one step further. In order to preserve energy for the body, companies have manipulated pure essential amino acids to be one step behind or one step beyond their original form. In other words, an entire metabolic step is eliminated, making it more bioavailable for the body. Ultimately, there can be enhanced therapeutic benefits with active forms of amino acids. Examples of these are discussed below.

In Appendix A, you will find a listing of potential therapeutic doses for specific amino acids. Although most amino acids are available at your local health food store, it is advisable to consult with a practitioner who is educated in nutrition.

Ornithine

Ornithine is manufactured when arginine is metabolized during the production of urea. Ornithine is often used by bodybuilders to enhance muscle-building capabilities and to increase lean body mass. Because of its ability to assist in muscle building, studies have shown ornithine to be effective for individuals posthospitalization, post-surgery, or following burns.

In one study of individuals with severe burns, supplementation with 10–30 grams of ornithine decreased hospital stays and increased wound healing.

L-Carnitine

This amino acid is made in the body from lysine and methionine. It is considered a conditionally essential amino acid. The main action of this amino acid is to transport fatty acids into the mitochondria, the cell responsible for making energy in our bodies. Here, the cell is required to turn fat into energy.

Therapeutically, L-carnitine has shown promising results in improving multiple parameters associated with heart disease. In one study of patients with high blood pressure and diabetes, L-carnitine was given for forty-five weeks. Following the study, both arrhythmias and abnormal heart functioning decreased significantly.

Several double-blind studies have demonstrated that L-carnitine also has significant benefits for individuals with angina because it improves circulation to the extremities. Angina is a condition that may lead to a heart attack.

In individuals with anorexia, L-carnitine has improved mental symptoms and decreased healing time. Other studies show L-carnitine to be effective in helping people with chronic obstructive pulmonary disease. One study showed that, after only four weeks, patients were able to breathe easier while exercising.

Studies of L-carnitine and athletic performance show mixed results. L-carnitine does appear to decrease muscle soreness following athletic activity, but it fails to actually improve performance.

Taurine

Taurine, like glutamine, is considered a conditionally essential amino acid, essential only when the body is stressed, such as with burns or injury. Taurine does not combine with other amino acids to form proteins; instead, it remains free in many tissues. Over 50 percent of taurine in the body is found in heart tissue. It is also a main component of bile acid, and is found in the retina and in neutrophils.

Vegans consume virtually no taurine in their diet, as it is found mainly in meats and fish protein. However, taurine can be produced from the amino acid cysteine in the presence of the cofactor vitamin B_6. If either cysteine or vitamin B_6 is absent, then taurine is deficient in the diet and should be supplemented. Taurine is essential for infants as they cannot make it themselves. They can receive enough either through breast milk, which is high in taurine, or through most infant formulas.

Taurine has been studied widely in various conditions that affect the heart. Taurine helps maintain the heart's intracellular calcium levels, which ultimately protects heart muscle. Taurine has positive inotropic effects, making it valuable for lowering blood pressure. It is also capable of lowering cholesterol levels and preventing cardiac arrhythmias.

Taurine has a unique ability as an amino acid to function as an antioxidant. It has demonstrated an ability to inhibit neutrophil bursting and subsequent oxidative stress, which can damage heart tissue. Because of this mechanism, taurine has been found to be beneficial in congestive heart failure.

Because of the high taurine concentration found in retinal tissue, taurine supplementation has been found to be useful in treating retinal degeneration and retinitis pigmentosa. Therapeutic effects are in part due to taurine's antioxidant properties. It also appears to regulate osmotic pressure in the eyes and inhibit lipid peroxidation.

Taurine, and a synthetic version of taurine called acamprosate, have proven to be very useful in the treatment of alcoholism and alcohol withdrawal. In one study, a dose of 1 gram taken three times daily during the withdrawal phase greatly reduced psychotic episodes. Also, individuals taking taurine were less likely to relapse.

Taurine has demonstrated therapeutic benefits in the treatment of diabetes, hepatitis, cystic fibrosis, and Alzheimer's disease.

SHOPPING FOR THE RIGHT PROTEIN SUPPLEMENT

Many people like to start their day with a protein shake or smoothie. It can be a good source of protein that gives you an energy boost, and it's a bit lighter than two eggs and bacon. The following information will help guide you to determine which type of complete protein supplementation is right for you. First choose the raw material—whey, soy, or rice—that best suits your health needs, then read the appropriate sections below.

Which Whey Supplement Is Right for You?

Shopping for a whey protein supplement can be a bit confusing. There are four types of commercially available whey proteins:

- Whey protein isolate

- Whey protein concentrate

- Hydrolyzed whey protein

- Undenatured whey protein concentrate

For each of these products, whey is processed in a unique way, resulting in a different protein concentration, as well as a different fat, lactose, and mineral content. In the isolate form, there is little to no fat, lactose, or mineral content, but it is high in pure protein. Whey protein concentration is most commonly available as 80 percent protein concentration with a small amount of fat, lactose, and minerals present. Hydrolyzed whey is often the least allergenic, due to the way the proteins are processed. Undenatured whey often has the highest concentration of immunoglobulins and lactoferrin, making it the best form for enhancing immunity. Undenatured whey concentrates are the least processed of the whey supplements.

During the processing of protein isolates—and this goes for any type of protein: whey, soy, or rice—the product is obtained by heating the protein to a high temperature. When these proteins are brought above 140 degrees Fahrenheit, a denaturing process begins. When a protein is denatured, it loses its native protein structure, and ultimately, its health benefit. Products that have undenatured protein components are generally more expensive and have more immune-potentiating effects. Whey products that have been heated above 140 degrees still have an adequate amino acid profile and can be used as a protein source; however, many of the important whey proteins such as lactoferrin and immunoglobulins are diminished.

In any concentrate form, manufacturers have the ability to manipulate protein concentration. As protein concentration increases, fat, lactose, and mineral contents decrease. During the processing of most whey concentrates, lactose is removed by an ion-exchange process to make the product less allergenic.

Lactose
A type of sugar found in milk. Some people have intolerance to lactose, resulting in an upset stomach.

In order to determine which form of whey is best suited for you, you must first determine if you have any allergies or intolerance to dairy. Because lactose is often removed in whey supplements, they are often tolerated by individuals who cannot ordinarily consume milk.

Secondly, look at several products for variable protein, fat, and mineral content to find one that suits you best. Lastly, if you are anticipating immune-enhancing effects, find a product that is high in lactoferrin and immunoglobulins.

Which Soy Supplement Is Right for You?

The single most important factor in purchasing a soy protein supplement is finding one that is organic. Today, most soy products are genetically engineered. Genetically modified proteins often contain foreign proteins that are likely to be highly irritating to the digestive tract and immune system.

Organic
A standard that keeps agricultural products from being sprayed with pesticides, herbicides, or other chemicals.

Some soy protein isolates are processed with an alcohol extraction to remove the phytoestrogens. If you are concerned about the estrogen effect of soy but want to use a soy protein supplement, it would be best to purchase an isolate product. Soy products that have not had the phytoestrogens removed typically contain about 1.2 milligrams per gram of protein as genistein, and 0.5 milligrams per gram of protein as daidzein.

Whey versus Soy: Which Is Easier to Digest?

Whey protein concentrates are more easily digested than soy proteins. For many individuals, soy consumption can lead to poor digestion, including gas and heartburn. In a randomized, double-blind study of elderly women, whey proteins, when compared to casein proteins, exhibited higher post-meal levels of various plasma amino acids. Whey is considered a "fast protein." It does not coagulate under acidic conditions (as in the stomach) and rapidly enters the small intestine to be digested.

Whey versus Soy: What Does the Research Say?

Whey appears to be more protective than soy against tumor growth, according to a recent study. The American Academy of Cancer Research found that whey protein, compared to soy or casein protein, was more effective in preventing tumor development. Whey was twice as effective as soy in reducing both tumor incidence and multiplicity.

In addition, some studies demonstrate that soy may actually promote tumor growth in estrogen-sensitive cancers such as breast, prostate, ovarian, and uterine cancer. If you have one of these cancers, or are at high risk for developing them, it is advised that you do not use a soy protein supplement.

Which Rice Protein Supplement Is Right for You?

The biggest difference between rice proteins is the carbohydrate content. If you have chosen rice as a protein source because you have allergies, a lower-carbohydrate rice protein may best suit your needs. If your body is in recovery from surgery, chemotherapy, or other major injury that causes difficulty ingesting solid food, a higher-carbohydrate rice protein may be best.

Some rice proteins are made from genetically modified rice. It is speculated that this can seriously affect the health benefits received. Also, some rice proteins are modified by recombinant DNA techniques. As a consumer, to ensure quality of your product, you can always ask for processing information from the manufacturer.

Other things to consider about rice proteins are that they do not have a high mineral content compared to other types of protein supplements. Be sure not to use it as a multivitamin/mineral substitute. Additionally, rice protein should not be used as a substitute for food, as it is inadequate nutritionally.

Also, if you have been diagnosed as being gluten intolerant, some rice proteins may not be good for you. In the enzymatic processing of the protein, one of the enzymes is derived from barley, which is a gluten grain. This may or may not affect your digestive system, depending on the level of your sensitivity. Contact the manufacturer to determine if barley, or other gluten grains, have been used.

CHAPTER 7

PROTEIN AND POPULAR DIETS

Most Americans are heavier than their optimum weight. Being overweight often controls what we think of ourselves and affects our health directly. In an effort to control the obesity epidemic in this country, individuals find themselves experimenting with different fad diets.

New statistics state that obesity reached a record high in the fall of 2004, with 60 percent of American adults becoming obese. Metabolic syndrome, clinically defined as cardiovascular disease accompanied by blood sugar irregularities and obesity, is the most pressing public health issue we face today. As a result, we are constantly searching for dietary solutions.

Unfortunately, not all diets are good for us, especially if not approached under medical supervision. Quick weight loss should not be the goal of any weight-loss program. Weight lost rapidly almost never stays off. To make matters worse, most of the weight lost is water weight, resulting in dehydration.

WHERE ARE WE GETTING OUR FOOD?

In a 2002 study carried out by the U.S. Department of Agriculture, it was determined that refined sugars, grains, vegetable oils, and dairy made up 70.9 percent of energy in the United States food supply. In 1970, Americans spent about $6 billion on fast food; in 2001, they spent more than $110 billion. Americans now spend more money on fast food than on higher education, new cars, movies, books, magazines, newspapers, and music combined.

The nation's three largest beverage manufacturers, Coca-Cola, Pepsi, and Schweppes, are spending large sums of money on marketing to children. Currently, these three companies control 90.3 percent of the U.S. market. They are entering our children's schools, contributing millions of dollars annually to school programs that have received less federal funding in recent years. As a result, soda ads appear in the hallways at schools, on the insides of school buses, in school newspapers, and at every school sporting event.

American adults drink soda at an alarming rate of 56 gallons per person annually. The amount of soda a typical teenage boy drinks has gone from 7 ounces a day in 1978 to nearly three times that amount today, accounting for 10 percent of his caloric intake. A significant number of teenage boys drink five or more cans of soda a day. Each can contains the equivalent of 10 teaspoons of sugar. These are empty calories, with zero nutrition.

THE HIGH-PROTEIN DIETS

High-protein diets have become the latest of fad diets to sweep the nation and its health food industry. Since the late Robert Atkins set the stage decades ago, several variations of the low-carbohydrate, high-protein diet have emerged. This section will give you an understanding of various diets.

The Atkins Diet: What's All the Hype?

According to the Atkins Diet, an increase in carbohydrate consumption can set off the following cascade: 1) Glucose levels increase, which elevates insulin output; 2) Increased insulin causes glucose levels to drop, leading to food cravings;

and, 3) Excessive caloric intake leads to body-fat storage, particularly in the abdominal area.

Insulin is a hormone released from the pancreas in response to sugar or glucose in the diet. In a healthy cell, insulin helps the body convert glucose to energy. In a fat cell, glucose is stored as fat.

By severely restricting dietary carbohydrates, the body goes into ketosis; that is, the body experiences an abnormal increase in ketones, a by-product of fat metabolism. According to Robert Atkins, this metabolic pathway simply breaks down stored fat. When the diet is high in carbohydrates, the body prefers to use them as fuel, storing the leftovers as fat. However, when carbohydrates are restricted, the body must use fat for fuel.

How Does It Work?

There are four phases to the Atkins Diet. In every phase, proteins and fats are eaten liberally. Carbohydrate intake changes from phase to phase. During the introductory phase, the first two weeks, you are allowed 20 grams of carbohydrates, which is roughly 3 cups of salad vegetables. After that, carbohydrates are added back into the diet in 5-gram increments until weight loss stops.

Atkins refers to this point as the Critical Carbohydrate for Losing Level (CCLL). Every individual has their own carbohydrate threshold; however, the average CCLL appears to be between 35 to 40 grams of carbohydrates per day. This results in a continual weight loss of a pound per week for the average person.

The Bottom Line

- Eating out is no longer an issue. Most restaurants, including fast-food chains, offer low-carb options.

- A costly diet, as meat costs more than fruits and vegetables.

- Not a vegetarian-friendly diet.

- High in saturated fat.

Will the Weight Stay Off?

The weight will stay off if you restrict carbohydrates indefinitely. When you reintroduce potato chips, cookies, bread, and pasta, the pounds will return.

The South Beach Diet

This diet, developed by cardiologist Arthur Agatston, M.D., director of Mount Sinai Cardiac Prevention Center, was developed with the intention of promoting weight loss without compromising heart health. Unlike other low-carbohydrate diets, the South Beach Diet tries to keep saturated fats in check by favoring lean protein sources such as fish and chicken over bacon, cheeseburgers, and steak.

How Does It Work?

There are three phases to this diet. In phase one, carbohydrates are decreased dramatically in an effort to limit cravings. This phase lasts two weeks. Fruit is not allowed during phase one due to its carbohydrate content. Dr. Agatston states in his 2003 book *The South Beach Diet*, "... most obesity is simple. The faster the sugar and starches you eat are processed and absorbed into your bloodstream, the fatter you get."

The second phase keeps blood sugar in check by adding a limited amount of "good carbohydrates." Good carbohydrates include those that are slowly digested, such as whole grains, fruits, and vegetables. These foods are ranked according to their glycemic index. (See Appendix C, Glycemic Index Reference Guide.)

During week two, people tend to lose a

pound a week. At this time, carbohydrates can be added back slowly until you reach your goal weight.

The final phase of this diet is the moderate diet plan that you intend to keep. The goal is to no longer feel that you are dieting; rather, you have changed your eating habits and the new regimen has become a way of life.

Glycemic Index (GI)

Measures the amount of glucose released into the body two hours after eating. Foods with a lower GI, those that release sugar more slowly, are favored.

The Bottom Line

- No calorie counting, just a simple understanding of what you eat.

- Eating out has become easy.

- Moderate cost.

- Again, not very vegetarian friendly.

Will the Weight Stay Off?

The weight will stay off as long as you are committed to a carbohydrate-modified diet.

The Salmon and Salad Diet

This diet, initiated by Dr. Ronald Hoffman of the Hoffman Center in New York City, stresses the importance of eating a whole-foods diet. He places foods in three groups: foods to be emphasized, foods to be enjoyed in limited moderation, and foods to avoid. Eight glasses of water should be consumed daily, and herbal teas are allowed.

Foods to Be Emphasized

Olive oil and omega-3 fatty acids, such as those that come from fish, are allowed in unlimited amounts. He recommends diversifying fish intake and avoiding farm-raised and smoked fish, as nutritional value is often lower. You can also have unlimited legumes, low-starch vegetables, and lean protein from poultry and eggs.

Fresh vegetables are emphasized since they provide a natural source of antioxidants. Again, diversity is always best. Make sure to include leafy greens, such as kale, spinach, and chard, as well as vegetables from the cabbage family, such as broccoli and cauliflower.

Antioxidant

A chemical or other agent that prevents oxidation. Oxidation occurs when a fatty molecule combines with an oxygen molecule, causing tissue damage or rancidity in food.

Salads and sprouts can be eaten in unlimited amounts, but salad dressings should be modified. Use foods such as olive oil, vinegar, lemon juice, garlic, or sesame oil to dress your salad.

Enjoy in Healthful Moderation

Dr. Hoffman suggests consuming no flour products but does allow limited whole grains, such as brown rice, quinoa, millet, rolled oats, buckwheat, and amaranth. Four ounces of whole grains are allowed per day. By eating whole grains instead of bread or pasta, it is easier to keep the glycemic index low.

Two ounces of nuts or nut butters a day are allowed. This includes sesame seeds, pumpkin seeds, almonds, hazelnuts, walnuts, and sunflower seeds. Make sure they are unsalted and raw, or roasted.

Corn, potatoes (not French fries), sweet potato, winter squash, carrots, and beets should be limited to two or three servings a week because of their high carbohydrate content.

Foods to Avoid

No unrefined sugar or artificial sweeteners are allowed on this diet, but that does not include fresh fruit. You can have one piece of fresh fruit daily. No hydrogenated or trans fats are to be consumed. Red meat and pork is optional, although commercially raised meats should be avoided. White rice and all flour products should be avoided, including breaded and fried foods.

The Bottom Line

- A healthy diet based on whole food.

- Moderate cost.

- Not a fast-food-friendly diet, but most restaurants are accommodating.

Will the Weight Stay Off?

The weight will stay off if you continue to eat whole foods. When you slip back to a diet with processed foods, the pounds will likely return.

The Zone Diet

The Zone Diet was created in 1995 by Dr. Barry Sears, Ph.D., to enhance the body's ability to burn fat and keep hunger away. An added selling point was that athletes using this diet could reach maximum performance levels. The key to this diet is attaining an accurate amount of protein, carbohydrates, and fats at each meal, allowing your body to reach a metabolic zone.

How Does It Work?

The nutrition ratio that needs to be attained in each meal is: 40 percent carbohydrate, 30 percent fat, and 30 percent protein. Food has to be eaten at precise times and is divided into three "zone friendly" meals and two "zone friendly" snacks. Dr. Sears believes that by eating the right food combination at a particular time, the body can keep hormones such as insulin in balance.

The Bottom Line

- It isn't easy. It takes a lot of dedication to count grams of each food for every meal.

- Eating out is a bit difficult. Restaurants aren't as menu friendly with this diet.

- Average cost.

- More vegetarian friendly.

Will the Weight Stay Off?

The goal here isn't weight loss so much as achieving the optimal ratio of body fat and maintaining it. It may take a lifetime for some.

THE MEAT-FREE DIETS

At the other end of the spectrum, opposite the high-protein dieters, are individuals who limit their intake of animal products. With animal proteins limited, or completely eliminated, adequate food combining to ensure a complete variety of all amino acids is difficult, but an absolute necessity. It is not unusual to find nutrient or even protein deficiencies in some individuals.

Vegetarian

Vegetarianism has a long history and may still be considered the most common type of diet on the planet. Even in the United States, vegetarianism was the predominant diet until the turn of century when beef consumption was on the rise. For many, it is a diet of necessity due to cultural, religious, and even spiritual beliefs. In some cultures, vegetarianism may be the only available option. Or the expense of animal products may be prohibitive.

A vegetarian diet is one that includes little to no animal products. Some vegetarians do include eggs and dairy in their diet, but for the most part vegetarians restrict meat, fish, and poultry. A lacto-ovo-vegetarian is a vegetarian who eats the byproducts of chickens and cows: eggs and milk products such as cheese and yogurt. Some vegetarians are "lacto" and not "ovo" because they do not feel comfortable eating unborn chickens, but will consume dairy products.

In the past few decades, vegetarianism has

become popular again. In general, it has been speculated that vegetarians have lower rates of heart disease, obesity, and cancer. The American Heart Association endorses this diet, as does the American Cancer Society.

Vegetarians tend to have lower cholesterol and triglyceride levels, which, if elevated, can contribute to heart disease and, ultimately, metabolic syndrome. Vegetarians consume lower amounts of protein and saturated fat, which are normally found in animal products. It has been suggested that saturated fat may contribute to heart disease, as well.

Vegan

Veganism is the most pure form of vegetarianism. There are absolutely no animal products allowed in this diet. The only foods that can be consumed are vegetables, fruits, legumes, grains, nuts, and seeds. Vegans tend to weigh less than the average person and are often underweight. Compared to a dairy- and/or egg-eating vegetarian, a vegan will almost always have lower cholesterol and triglyceride levels.

This diet is not recommended for children or pregnant or nursing women. It is very difficult to get the right amount of nutrition, particularly proteins, during times of increased growth. Without adequate nutrition, growth and development may be stunted, along with impairments to the nervous and immune systems.

Can You Get Enough Protein in a Meat-Free Diet?

Because most vegetarian foods are not complete proteins, it is not unusual to find some amino acid imbalances. Vegetable proteins tend to be low in one or two of the essential amino acids. Grains, legumes, seeds, nuts, and vegetables are all examples of incomplete proteins. For example, beans are deficient in lysine while rice, which has sufficient lysine, is low in methionine.

Food combining can be an important part of maintaining a healthy vegetarian diet. The following are different food combinations that can provide complete proteins:

- Grains and legumes: rice and lentils; wheat and peas; bean burritos

- Seeds/nuts and legumes: garbanzo beans and sesame (hummus); tofu and sesame

- Grains and milk/eggs: quiche; rice and eggs; French toast; lasagna

- Vegetables and milk/eggs: cream soup; vegetables with eggs; salad with egg; omelet

In general, both vegetarians and vegans can get enough protein if they are diligent with their diet. It is extremely important to make sure there are adequate legumes, nuts, and seeds, which is where most of the protein in their diet will come from.

Are There Any Health Risks Associated with a Meat-Free Diet?

Many vegetarians often find that they consume too many carbohydrates. This may in part be due to a diet with inadequate protein intake, resulting in carbohydrate cravings. Other reasons for increased carbohydrate intake include lack of diversity in the diet and a diet of convenience, that is, eating what is available. More often than not, fast food and vending machines offer higher-carbohydrate options.

A diet with excess carbohydrates, combined with a sedentary lifestyle, can lead to obesity. It is not unusual to find an individual who, after ten years of vegetarianism, has an elevated body mass index (BMI). Cholesterol and triglycerides may be low in vegetarians, but being obese is just as much of a risk factor as having high cholesterol and triglycerides. The solution to this is ultimately making sure you get enough exercise.

Body Mass Index (BMI)
A measurement of body fat based on height and weight. The result indicates one's risk of disease.

One of the most important health issues for vegetarians, particularly vegans, is a reduced iron and vitamin B_{12} intake, which can result in increased levels of anemia. Both iron and B_{12} are found in meat, poultry, and fish. Iron can be obtained from nonanimal sources in small amounts. It is hotly debated as to whether or not vitamin B_{12} is available from nonanimal sources. Some say that brewer's yeast can provide B_{12}.

Nonanimal Sources of Iron

- Amaranth
- Lentils
- Molasses
- Seaweed
- Tofu

Iron and vitamin B_{12} should be supplemented if either is found to be low. Oftentimes, B_{12} intramuscular injections need to be administered in order to maintain adequate amounts. A vitamin B_{12} deficiency can lead to poor metabolism of protein, fats, and carbohydrates, problems of the nervous system, and problems with red blood cell counts.

In addition to iron and B_{12} deficiency, vegetarians, especially vegans, often have mineral deficiencies. This is largely because a vegetarian diet often lacks the fat-soluble catalyst found in animal products that is needed for mineral absorption. Furthermore, phytates, which are found in grains and soy, may block absorption of minerals such as calcium, zinc, copper, and magnesium.

Zinc, calcium, and other minerals from animal

sources are usually more absorbable when they come from animal sources. In humans, research has shown that zinc deficiency can lead to learning disabilities and mental retardation. In men, zinc deficiency can cause infertility. Again, it can't be stressed enough that a well-rounded diet, including animal products in moderation, is essential for normal growth and development of children.

What Are the Health Benefits of a Vegetarian Diet?

In addition to protecting against heart disease and cancer, as previously mentioned, a vegetarian diet can prove therapeutic when used for a designated period of time. In general, a diet that consists of meat tends to be more acidic and more "inflammatory." Arachidonic acid is a by-product that comes from the digestion of animal fats. It has a tendency to lead the body down inflammatory pathways.

In many cultures throughout history, individuals have performed "cleanses" and fasts. A fast, which is a complete elimination of food, is different from a cleanse, which limits certain foods for a period of time. Often during a cleanse, meats and other animal products are eliminated from the diet to allow the body a "rest period" from metabolizing protein. This can ultimately decrease inflammation, cholesterol, and triglycerides.

As you learned in the previous chapters, diversified protein in the diet is essential to maintaining all physiologic functions in the body. Therefore, daily, moderate protein intake is important. Fasts should be done for a brief amount of time, under strict medical supervision. Cleanses can be done regularly, either one day a week, monthly, or seasonally.

When the body is in an acute state of a disease process, it is a good idea to avoid animal fats and proteins until your body has fully recovered. Times when this might be beneficial are: after an acute sports- or job-related injury, after surgery, and if you have inflammatory arthritis, a cold, or the flu. Because protein is necessary for growth and maintenance of healthy body tissue, protein should be added back into the diet when inflammation has begun to subside.

BENEFICIAL BEHAVIOR PATTERNS FOR ACHIEVING OPTIMAL WEIGHT

The following are ten basic guidelines to help you achieve your optimal weight:

1. Drink eight to ten glasses of water a day, but not with meals.

2. Practice eating only when hungry.

3. Decrease or avoid alcohol and caffeine consumption.

4. Shop for food after you have eaten, not when hungry.

5. Eat your bigger meals earlier in the day for optimal calorie utilization.

6. Get support from family and friends to encourage you and to share healthy eating habits with you.

7. Wait ten to fifteen minutes before eating second helpings; your hunger will subside.

8. Plan meals and food choices ahead of time.

9. Eat slowly and chew your food well. Never eat in front of the television.

10. Educate yourself about healthy food choices. Attend cooking classes and nutrition workshops.

CHAPTER 8

PROS AND CONS OF A HIGH-PROTEIN DIET

High-protein diets have created quite a bit of controversy in recent years. The bottom line for most individuals is *you can lose weight on these diets*. While several doctors feel encouraged by the amount of weight loss and the improvement in insulin sensitivity, many feel that the high-protein diets emphasize far too much saturated fat, contributing to further heart disease, increased cholesterol levels, and a higher risk of developing cancer, particularly colon, breast, and prostate cancer.

Insulin Sensitivity
A condition that occurs when the body's cells lose their ability to respond to insulin secretion. This results in increased blood sugar and the development of diabetes.

A good deal of time and money has gone into researching these diets, mostly because of the obesity epidemic. Studies are suggesting that, in the short term, high-protein diets have a favorable effect on cholesterol and triglycerides levels, particularly high-density lipoprotein (HDL). They can also be extremely important when short-term weight loss is required. However, with the enormous amount of saturated fat ingested, nutritionists are concerned about the long-term health effects, which are currently being studied.

High-density Lipoprotein (HDL)
"Good" cholesterol; transports cholesterol from the tissues to the liver where it is broken down. Optimal range is 45–65 mg per deciliter.

As mentioned in Chapter 1, the ultimate problem some people have with high-protein diets may not be the increase in protein but rather the increase in total calories, total fat, and saturated fat that can accompany consumption of animal protein.

WHAT'S WRONG WITH LOSING WEIGHT THIS WAY?

Dietary protein requirements are influenced by carbohydrate consumption. When carbohydrate intake is low, amino acids are deaminated, or broken down, to provide a carbon skeleton to synthesize glucose to be used as fuel. As mentioned in Chapter 1, the brain and heart absolutely need glucose to function. If carbohydrate intake is less than 150 grams per day, substantial amounts of protein are utilized to make precursors for gluconeogenesis.

Gluconeogenesis
The chemical transformation of amino acids into glucose or glycogen. Eighteen amino acids have the chemical structure that allows for conversion.

After relying on a high-protein diet for an extended period of time, many individuals can begin to feel debilitated. Our bodies do not store extra amino acids, unlike fat, which many of us have plenty of. Our only protein stores are found in our muscles. When the body needs energy or fuel, after fat stores are depleted, we begin to eat away at our muscles. This can leave us feeling exhausted and weak. Exercise may become harder to perform, making it difficult to tone our muscles following weight loss.

Depletion of Food Stores in the Body Tissues

Because the body normally uses carbohydrates and fats for energy before it uses protein stores, carbohydrates and fats are called "protein sparers." The quantity of carbohydrate stored in the body is only a few hundred grams, mainly as glycogen in the liver and muscles, and can provide enough energy for approximately half a day. On the first day of a high-protein, low-carbohydrate diet, the body utilizes all available carbohydrate stores. The effects that follow include progressive depletion of tissue fat and protein.

Fat becomes the prime source of energy for the body, which for many is the goal of this diet. In a "normal person," there is 100 times more fat energy stored in the body than carbohydrate energy. The rate of fat utilization continues unabated until fat stores run out, which, for most of us, will never happen.

Protein undergoes three phases of energy utilization. The first phase involves rapid utilization, then a more gradual utilization, and then a final period of rapid utilization before the body is ultimately depleted of resources.

The protein used in the first phase is easily mobilized protein for direct metabolism or for conversion to glucose (gluconeogenesis), which will then be metabolized to nourish the brain. After the readily mobile stores have been depleted, because of physiologic stress on the body, the body's remaining protein becomes more difficult to remove. In the initial phase of a high-protein diet, people in general feel very good, some may even call it euphoric. The body is working with leaner conditions, in an efficient metabolic state.

The second phase of protein depletion begins around the time in the diet when individuals report feeling weak and exhausted and experience an inability to continue exercise. The rate of gluconeogenesis begins to decrease to about one-fifth its previous rate, making the body starving for glucose. The lessened availability of glucose initiates a series of events that allows fat to be utilized at an excessive rate, creating ketone bodies (leading to ketosis).

Ketone bodies, like glucose, cross the blood-brain barrier and can be used by the brain and heart. At this point in the diet, about two-thirds of the brain's energy is derived from ketone bodies, principally from beta-hydroxybutyrate. This can often lead to feeling foggy-headed or light-headed. Some have reported feeling more confused than usual.

Ultimately, if the diet is continued and fat stores are depleted, protein utilization becomes rapid again. Protein is the main source of energy. At this point in the diet, individuals usually suffer from muscle wasting and overall deterioration of skin integrity. Oftentimes, the face takes on a grayish hue.

Ketosis

Some high-protein, low-carbohydrate diets are designed to put the body in ketosis. After the body is depleted of carbohydrate energy stores, the body searches for a new source of glucose—ketone bodies. Ketone bodies are made from fatty acids, which are a metabolic byproduct of fat degradation.

An increase in ketone bodies can result in a shift in the body's acid-base balance. Studies do suggest that when the body is in metabolic acidosis for a prolonged period of time, low blood phosphate levels can occur. This can ultimately lead to resorption of calcium from bone, putting individuals at increased risk of osteoporosis There is also an increased tendency to form kidney stones.

Cancer Causing?

As mentioned earlier, it has been well documented that a diet high in saturated fat is a risk factor for some cancers. High-protein, low-carbohydrate diets often tend to be low in vegetable and fruit intake. Fruits and vegetables are naturally high in fiber. When fiber is reduced in the body, regular bowel function is often limited. Several clinical trials have proven that high-fiber diets can have a significant impact of reducing the symptoms of constipation, diarrhea, and general bowel irritability.

In a study analyzing long-term health effects of people on the Atkins Diet, it was discovered that during the initial phases of the diet, only 2 grams of fiber were consumed daily. During the maintenance phase, up to 18 grams of fiber were eaten daily. The Institute of Medicine recommends 14 grams of fiber per 1,000 kilocalories, which is equivalent to 28–42 grams per day for the average adult.

High-protein foods tend to be low in a group of vitamins and minerals considered to have antioxidant properties. To make matters worse, these foods also tend to have a pro-oxidative effect in the body. On the other hand, fruits and vegetables, which are limited in many phases of high-protein diets, are extremely high in antioxidants. Studies have established that antioxidants are beneficial in preventing certain cancers and heart disease.

The Kidneys

In a six-month trial at Duke University studying the effects of a high-protein diet, one-fifth of participants reported having some type of kidney problem. Complaints included reduced kidney function, increased kidney stone formation, and increased tendency to develop kidney infections.

It is clear that eating protein forces the kidneys to work harder. Protein is deaminated, or broken down, in the kidneys as well as the liver. The byproducts, if not eliminated readily by the kidneys, can cause significant tissue damage.

In addition, protein ingestion increases renal acid secretion and calcium resorption from bone, while reducing renal calcium resorption. Also, eating animal proteins, which are high in purines, tends to result in the intracellular production of uric acid. When uric acid builds up, especially in an existing acidic environment, it can both form uric acid stones and decrease the solubility of calcium oxalate, making some individuals at greater risk for calcium stones.

Osteoporosis

Osteoporosis is a disorder characterized by abnormal rates of bone fracture, particularly in the hip and spine. It usually occurs in the elderly unless induced by medications such as long-term steroid therapy. Ninety-nine percent of the body's calcium is stored in the bones; therefore, there is a direct relationship between calcium metabolism and bone density.

The link between osteoporosis and a high-protein diet is suggested by the following. Elevated protein intake is said to increase urinary calcium loss, increasing the risk for fracture. When carbohydrates are limited and ketosis is allowed to occur, the body's increased acidic state magnifies the effects of calcium loss.

Bad Breath

Often, people on a high-protein, low-carbohydrate diet report symptoms of bad breath or having a funny taste in their mouth. This usually happens when ketosis occurs. In a six-month trial out of Duke University, problems with bad breath were reported in 63 percent of patients on a high-protein diet.

When fatty acids are the primary source of energy and carbohydrates are heavily restricted, part of the free-fat particles can't be metabolized, and it builds up outside the cell. These particles are converted to ketones, and unused ketones are excreted in the urine and expired air, resulting in acetone-smelling breath.

Toxic Fat?

Additionally, with a diet high in fat, you run the risk of consuming a large amount of toxins. Toxins bio-accumulate in the fatty tissue of animals, which in turn are consumed when you eat products such as eggs, dairy, and meat. One way to avoid such toxins is to eat organic food, and eggs from free-range chickens. Organic food is upheld to a standard such that there is no herbicide or pesticide application. In addition, organic animal products do not contain any antibiotics or growth hormones.

Toxins Found in Nonorganic Animal Products

- Heavy metals
- Herbicides
- PCBs
- Pesticides

By avoiding animal products with antibiotics and growth hormones, you create a healthier ecosystem for your body. Ingesting animal products that are contaminated with antibiotics can decrease your body's immunity. Animal products containing growth hormones can affect your body's natural hormone systems. Scientific studies are continually investigating the role of bovine growth hormones in the development of hormone-sensitive cancers such as breast and prostate cancer.

In general, the meat, eggs, and dairy products found in a standard supermarket have significantly less nutrition than they did just a few decades ago. Modern cattle-raising techniques often include the use of steroid hormones to make meat more tender. Many cattle that supply steak and ground beef to the American market have never seen the open range. Diseased animals routinely pass inspection and find their way into the food supply.

Chickens are often raised in crowded pens and are forced to lie under artificial light both by day and night. Chickens and cows are often fed animal feed containing animal parts, which is not normal to their diet. Infection often results, which in turn results in the use of antibiotics.

THE GOOD NEWS!

Not all high-protein, low-carbohydrate diets are as extreme as the Atkins Diet. If you are eating a high-protein diet filled with fresh fruits and vegetables but limited bread, pasta, or cereals, it is likely you will obtain plenty of antioxidants and fiber. You will not reach the point of protein utilization when muscle protein stores are depleted. And you will lose weight.

You can eat a high-protein diet that is not high in saturated fat by consuming a good amount of fish, nuts, nut butters, and lean meats such as poultry. There are also healthy ways to reduce carbohydrates in the body; they require being diligent about limiting intake and choosing whole foods over processed foods.

One of the single most important aspects of any diet is changing your eating habits. If for six weeks you cook your own meals and eat whole foods—fresh fruits, vegetables, and lean meats— you will lose weight. If after the six-week period you go back to your old ways—eating out, eating processed foods—you will put weight back on. The solution is to find time to cook and eat healthfully. It is truly the only way to stay fit and strong.

Whole Foods

- Dairy
- Eggs
- Fresh fruit
- Fresh vegetables
- Legumes

- Meat, fish, poultry
- Sea vegetables
- Seeds and nuts
- Whole grains

ARE "LOW-CARB" FOODS REALLY GOOD FOR ME?

Like any other health craze, the health food industry has taken advantage of our desire to lose weight and keep it off. The bottom line is "low-carb" foods are not whole foods. They are processed, packaged foods. Additionally, they tend to be higher in calories than unprocessed foods. If you eat too many "low-carb" foods, you will put weight back on, and quickly. Don't assume that because it is in the health food store, it is good for you.

HELP! WHAT IS THE ANSWER?

The answer for many is a controlled-carbohydrate diet. Most important, do not increase total caloric intake when shifting to a controlled-carbohydrate diet. You will need to determine what combination of the diets mentioned in this book is right for you. The combination will differ for every individual.

A controlled-carbohydrate diet, simply put, means avoiding breads, pastas, and other flour products *in excess.* Think moderation! First try decreasing intake to one or two servings of carbohydrate a day. A serving might include one slice of bread instead of two, so try an open-faced sandwich.

Also, be mindful of serving sizes. Don't super size. A simple 3- to 5-ounce serving of protein is all that is required per meal. There is no need to eat a burger or steak that is 8 or even 16 ounces!

If we all ate this way, the planet and ecosystem would surely pay the price.

When you eat organic animal products, the animals are usually contained under more humane conditions and allowed to feed and graze as animals should. Oftentimes, nonorganic but free-range products are also antibiotic- and hormone-free. Don't hesitate to ask your local supermarket butcher these important questions.

Because dieting can be stressful, many fear a lunch date with a friend or coworker. You can still go to your favorite deli for lunch, as long as you avoid the potato chips that come with your sandwich. Eat only half of the bread (one slice). Wash it down with some water, not juice or a soda, which only provide your body with empty calories. You can always order a salad with some variety of protein to top it off: grilled chicken breast or fish, hard-boiled egg or tofu. Be sure to use a vinegar-based salad dressing and avoid the creamy ones. Vinegar aids the digestive process.

Always make sure you have some form of protein with each of your three major meals. This will ultimately prevent food cravings and munchie attacks between meals. Keep healthy snacks in your car if you spend a lot of time on the road, or in your desk at work. This way, you are not spending your money at vending machines on food that you will regret eating later.

Drink plenty of water. When losing weight, it is very important to stay adequately hydrated. Your liver and kidneys both rely on water to assist in elimination of metabolic byproducts.

The following are some helpful tips to follow when making smart, healthy food choices:

- Eggs are the best source of complete protein for the body. Buy eggs from pasture-fed (free-range) chickens. These eggs tend to be brown and are found in all health food stores and now in almost every standard grocery store.

- Make a habit of eating fish, particularly cold-water, deep-sea fish. They are rich in omega-3 fatty acids, fat-soluble vitamins, and many important minerals.

- Consume dairy products in moderation. Use organic when possible, but at the very least make sure your milk products do not contain bovine growth hormones or antibiotics. If you can obtain raw, unpasteurized dairy products, these are most ideal for protein utilization.

- Eat plenty of fresh fruits and vegetables daily! Again, organic is best, but eating them at all is most important!

- Avoid processed meats that are preserved with nitrites, nitrates, and other preservatives. They only impede the road to health. Both bacon and sausage are available without these preservatives.

- Eat charcoal-grilled and smoked meats in moderation, as they contain chemicals called polycyclic aromatic hydrocarbons, which have been proven to cause cancer in laboratory animals.

CONCLUSION

If you took protein for granted before you read this book, you certainly don't now. As you have learned, protein is a fundamental life force! Every system in the body relies on protein for energy, enzyme production, as building blocks, and for basic metabolism.

To reach optimal health and wellness, it is important to practice dietary diversity. The value of protein to the body is partially dependant on vitamins, minerals, fats, and other compounds that assist in protein delivery and assimilation. To maximize the benefits of a healthy diet, it is important to eat a variety of high-quality proteins, as well as multiple fruits, vegetables, and whole grains, daily.

The biochemistry underlying the impact of protein, fat, and carbohydrates on the body is relatively static. Yet we are still bombarded with the newest and coolest diets for weight loss, vitality, and disease prevention. Protein is the centerpiece of most of the recent popular diets.

Before committing to any new diet, it is helpful to understand the basic nutritional biochemistry the diet provides; that is, the diet's protein and amino acid content and how that affects the body in health and disease. The *User's Guide to Protein and Amino Acids* has given you the tools you need to evaluate various diets.

There is no one optimal diet for everyone. We are all individuals carrying our own genetic background, allergies, and sensitivities. But one fact remains constant: the body requires protein. Now you must take the first step by choosing sources that will be best for you.

Knowledge is power and by understanding proteins and amino acids you will now be able to separate fad from fact when confronted with the latest and greatest diet. You can approach the protein supplement aisle at the store with confidence that you are purchasing what is right for you.

Your understanding of individual amino acids will help you use them to maintain health, as well as support the body during disease. However, it is important to consult with a healthcare practitioner whenever there is serious illness or you are considering high-dose or long-term therapy.

Ultimately, you are responsible for what you eat. Be mindful when making dietary choices regarding protein consumption. The *User's Guide to Protein and Amino Acids* by no means contains the absolute answers for every individual. It does, however, provide the information needed to guide you through diet and supplement decisions about protein.

AMINO ACID DOSING RECOMMENDATIONS

This is a general guide to be used to find suggested doses only. Individual amino acid doses vary for different conditions. For optimal results, consult with your health practitioner. (Only those amino acids that are used therapeutically are included here.)

Alanine
Natural sources: Meat, poultry, fish, eggs, dairy
Dose: 0.5–1 gram per day

Arginine
Natural sources: Dairy, meat, poultry, fish; nuts and chocolate also have fairly high amounts
Dose: 2–30 grams per day

Cysteine
Natural sources: Yogurt, poultry, eggs
Dose: In the form of N-acetyl cysteine: beginning at 500 milligrams per day, working up to 5 grams per day

Glutamine
Natural sources: Fish, meat, beans, dairy
Dose: 6–12 grams per day

Glycine
Natural sources: Fish, meat, beans, dairy
Dose: 500 milligrams to several grams per day

Histidine
Natural sources: Dairy, meat, poultry, fish
Dose: 1–8 grams per day, based on human research

Isoleucine
Natural sources: Dairy, red meat, whey protein
Dose: 2 grams per day

L-Carnitine
Natural sources: Dark turkey meat, red meat
Dose: 1–2 grams per day; 2 grams appear to
be optimal

Leucine
Natural sources: Dairy, red meat, whey protein
Dose: 5 grams per day

Lysine
Natural sources: Brewer's yeast, legumes, dairy,
fish, meat
Dose: 1–3 grams per day

Methionine
Natural sources: Eggs, sunflower seeds, meat,
fish, dairy
Dose: Most adults require 800–1,000 milligrams
of methionine a day, which is easily exceeded
by the diet. Doses of 7 grams per day have
been reported.

Ornithine
Natural sources: Meat, fish, dairy, eggs
Dose: 5–10 grams per day, based on human
research; sometimes used in combination with
arginine

Phenylalanine
Natural sources: Dairy, chicken, fish, soy, and
virtually every other protein-containing food
Dose: 1–6 grams per day

Taurine
Natural sources: Meat, fish
Dose: 1–2 grams per day

Tryptophan
Natural sources: Dairy, peanuts, turkey
Dose: 1–3 grams per day

Tyrosine
Natural sources: Dairy, meat, fish, wheat, oats
Dose: Most people should not supplement it;
however, a few conditions are treated with
7 grams per day.

Valine
Natural sources: Dairy, red meat, whey protein
Dose: 4 grams per day

A COMPARISON OF AMINO ACID CONTENT

LACTOFERRIN FROM WHEY (COW'S MILK) VS. HUMAN MILK

	Lactoferrin Residue from Cow's Milk	Lactoferrin Residue from Human Milk
Alanine	67	63
Arginine	39	43
Asparagine	29	33
Aspartic acid	36	38
Cysteine	34	32
Glutamic acid	40	42
Glutamine	29	27
Glycine	48	54
Histidine	9	9
Isoleucine	15	16
Leucine	65	58
Lysine	54	46
Methionine	4	5
Phenylalanine	27	30
Proline	30	35
Serine	45	50
Threonine	36	31
Tryptophan	13	10
Tyrosine	22	21
Valine	47	48

As you can see, in this table whey and human milk have comparable amino acid ratios. Human milk helps build a healthy immune system in a breastfed child. It is near impossible to create a substitute for mother's milk; however, whey can provide a similar chemical makeup.

Table adapted from Pierce A., Colavizza D., Benaissa M., et al. Molecular cloning and sequence analysis of bovine lactoferrin. Eur J Biochem 1991;177–184.

GLYCEMIC INDEX
REFERENCE GUIDE

The glycemic index (GI) refers to the amount of glucose released by foods within two hours of eating them. Foods with a higher glycemic index, greater than 50, release glucose into the bloodstream faster than do foods with a lower glycemic index. This information may be important when treating individuals with glucose metabolism disorders, including diabetes, metabolic syndrome, and hypoglycemia.

GI: 100
Glucose

GI: 80 to 90
Carrots
Corn flakes
Honey
Maltose
Parsnips
Potatoes (instant)
White bread

GI: 70 to 90
Bread (whole wheat)
Millet
Potatoes (fresh)
Rice (white)

GI: 60 to 90
Bananas
Muesli

Raisins
Rice (brown)
Shredded wheat

GI: 50 to 59
All-Bran
Buckwheat
Corn
Peas (frozen)
Potato chips
Spaghetti (white)
Sucrose
Yams

GI: 40 to 49
Beans (canned navy)
Oranges/orange juice
Peas (dried)
Potato (sweet)
Spaghetti
   (whole wheat)

GI: 30 to 39	**GI: 20 to 29**
Apples	Fructose
Black-eyed peas	Kidney beans
Butter beans	Lentils
Chickpeas	
Milk (whole and skim)	**GI: 10 to 19**
Tomato soup	Nuts
Vanilla ice cream	
Yogurt	

Note: All animal products, including meats, fish, eggs, and dairy are high-protein foods. Due to the low carbohydrate content, they all have a glycemic index of less than 50, suggesting the glucose levels enter gradually.

SELECTED
REFERENCES

Appel LJ, Moore TJ, Obarzanak E, et al. A clinical trial of the effects of dietary patterns on blood pressure. DASH Collaborative Research Group. *N Eng J Med* 1997;336:1117–1124.

Boirie Y, Dangin M, Gachon P, et al. Slow and fast dietary proteins differently modulate postprandial protein accretion. *Proc Natl Acad Sci USA* 1997;94: 14930–14935.

Bos C, Gaudichon C, Tome D. Nutritional and physiological criteria in the assessment of milk protein quality for humans. *J Am Coll Nutr* 2000;19:191S–205S.

Caruso I, et al. Double-blind study of 5 hydroxytryptophan versus placebo in the treatment of primary fibromyalgia syndrome. *J Int Med Res* 1990;18: 201–209.

Diet, Nutrition and the Prevention of Chronic Diseases. Report of a joint WHO/FAO expert consultation. WHO Technical Report Series 916, 2003.

Foster GD. A randomized trial of a low-carb diet for obesity. *N Engl J Med* 2003;348:2082–2090.

Gerrior S, Bente I. Nutrient content of the US food supply, 1909–1999: A summary report. USDA Center for Nutrition Policy and Promotion. Home Economics Research Report No. 55, 2002.

Griffiths RD. Outcome of critically ill patients after supplementation with glutamine. *Nutrition* 1997;13: 752–754.

Kimball SR, Jefferson LS. Control of protein synthesis by amino acid availability. *Curr Opin Clin Nutr Metab Care* 2002;5:63–67.

Lands LC, Grey YL, Smountas AA. Effect of supplementation with a cysteine donor on muscular performance. *J Appl Physiol* 1999;87:1381–1385.

Lemon P. Is increased dietary protein necessary for individuals with a physically active life? *Nutr Rev* 1996; 54:S169–175.

Marshall, K. Therapeutic applications of whey protein. *Altern Med Rev* 2004;9(2):136–156.

Marz R. *Medical Nutrition from Marz,* 2nd ed. Portland, OR: Omni Press, 2002.

Messina M, Persky V, Setchell K, Barnes S. Soy intake and cancer risk: a review of the in vitro and in vivo data. *Nutr Cancer* 1994;21:113–121.

Millward DJ, Pacy PJ. Postprandial protein utilization and protein quality assessment in man. *Clin Sci* 1995; 88:597–606.

Reddy ST, Wang CY, Sakhaee K, Brinkley L, Pak CY. Effect of low carbohydrate high protein diets on acid-base balance, stone forming propensity, and calcium metabolism. *Am J Kidney Dis* 2002;40:265–274.

Samaha FF. A low carbohydrate diet as compared with a low-fat diet in severe obesity. *N Engl J Med* 2003; 348:2074–2081.

Second International Symposium on the Role of Soy in Preventing and Treating Chronic Disease. Brussels, Belgium. September 15–18, 1996. Am *J Clin Nutr* 1998; 68: Suppl 1329S–1544S.

Sitrija V, Suvanpha R. Low protein diet and chronic renal failure in Buddhist monks. *BMJ* 1983;287: 469–471.

Smyth JF, Bowman A, Perren T, et al. Glutathione reduces the toxicity and improves quality of life of women diagnosed with ovarian cancer treated with cisplatin: results of a double-blind randomized trial. *Ann Oncol* 1997;8:569–573.

St Jeor ST, Howard BV, Prewitt TE, Bovee V, et al. Dietary protein and weight reduction: a statement for healthcare professionals from the Nutrition Committee of the Council on Nutrition, Physical Activity, and Metabolism of the American Heart Association. *Circulation* 2001;104:1869–1874.

Westman EC, Yancy WS, Edman JS, et al. Effect of 6-month adherence to a very low carbohydrate program. *Am J Med* 2002;113:30–36.

Yancy WS, Olsen MK, Guyton JR, Bakset RP, et al. A low carbohydrate, ketogenic diet versus a low fat diet to treat obesity and hyperlipidemia. *Ann Int Med* 2004; 140:769–777.

Young VR, Pellet PL. Plant proteins in relation to animal proteins and amino acid nutrition. *Am J Clin Nutr* 1994; 59 Suppl 1203S–1212S.

Zello GA, Wykes LF, Ball RO, et al. Recent advances in methods of assessing dietary amino acid requirements for adult humans. *J Nutr* 1995;125:2907–2915.

OTHER RESOURCES

American Association of Naturopathic Physicians (AANP)
3201 New Mexico Avenue, NW, Suite 350
Washington, D.C. 20016
1-866-538-2267
www.naturopathic.org
National organization with a find-a-doctor directory, for qualified doctors with nutritional expertise.

GreatLife Magazine
Consumer magazine with articles on vitamins, minerals, herbs, and foods.
Available for free at many health and natural food stores.

Let's Live Magazine
Consumer magazine with emphasis on the health benefits of vitamins, minerals, and herbs.
Customer service:
1-800-676-4333
P.O. Box 74908
Los Angeles, CA 90004
Subscriptions: 12 issues per year, $19.95 in the U.S.; $31.95 outside the U.S.

Physical Magazine
Magazine oriented to body builders and other serious athletes.
Customer service:
1-800-676-4333
P.O. Box 74908
Los Angeles, CA 90004

Subscriptions: 12 issues per year, $19.95 in the U.S.; $31.95 outside the U.S.

The Nutrition Reporter™ newsletter

Monthly newsletter that summarizes recent medical research on vitamins, minerals, and herbs.

Customer service:
P.O. Box 30246
Tucson, AZ 85751-0246
e-mail: jack@thenutritionreporter.com
www.nutritionreporter.com

Subscriptions: $26 per year (12 issues) in the U.S.; $32 U.S. or $48 CNC for Canada; $38 for other countries

Soybean Association of North America

1723 U Street, NW
Washington, D.C. 20009
202-986-5600

Weston A. Price Foundation

4200 Wisconsin Ave., NW
Washington, D.C. 20016
202-333-HEAL
WestonAPrice@msn.com

INDEX

Iron, 61
non-animal sources of, 61
Isoleucine, 13, 33, 78, 80

Ketone bodies, 67, 70
Ketosis, 67, 69
Kidneys, 68–69
Kwashiorkor, 7

Lactate dehydrogenase, 20
Lactoferrin, 22, 80–81
Lactose, 47
L-carnitine, 44, 78
L-dopa, 32, 38
Legumes, 60, 72
Lentils, 61
Leucine, 13, 33, 78, 80
Liver, 11, 20
Lysine, 13, 28–29, 44, 78, 80

Meal planning, 63
Meal timing, 63
Meat, 58–63, 72
grilled, 74
processed, 74
Meat-free diets, 58–63
heath risks, 60–62
Mechanical support, 17–18
Menopause, 24
Metabolic pathways, 19
Metabolism, 11
Metabolization of protein, 11
Metals, heavy, 35, 70
Methionine, 13, 29–31, 44, 78, 80
Milk products. *See* Dairy products.
Molasses, 61
Mount Sinai Cardiac Prevention Center, 54
Muscles, 43–44, 65
Myoglobin, 16

N-acetyl cysteine (NAC), 34
Natural killer (NK) cells, 37
Nerve generation and impulses, 19
Nervous sytem, 19
Net protein utilization. *See* NPU.
Niacinamide, 32
Nitric oxide, 39

Nitrogen, 4–6
sources, 4–5
Noradrenaline, 32
Norepinephrine. *See* Noradrenaline.
NPU, 5, 26
Nutrition, 36
Nutrition. *See* Diet.
Nutrition ratio, 57
Nutritional supplements. *See* Supplements.
Nuts, 60, 72

Obesity, 51–63, 64
Oils, olive, 55
Omega-3 fatty acids, 55, 74
Organic, 48, 70–71
Organic animal products, 73
Ornithine, 13, 43–44, 78
Osteoarthritis, 30
Osteoporosis, 69

Pancreas, 6
PCBs, 70
PEM, 7
Peptide bonds, 6, 9, 40
Pesticides, 70
pH balance. *See* Acid-alkaline balance.
Phenylalanine, 13, 32–33, 78, 80
Phytic acid, 26
Phytoestrogens, 25
PKU, 32–33, 38
Plasma, 20
Plasma enzymes, 19–20
Polypeptides, 10
Poultry, 72
Proline, 13, 80
Protein, 3–8, 9–14, 15–20, 21–27, 28–42, 43–50, 51–63, 64–74, 75–76, 77–79
body's role in making, 11–12
composition of, 9–14
deficiency, 7
definition, 3–8
depletion, 65–67
diets and, 51–63, 64–74
digesting, 5–6
dosages, 27

Printed in the USA
CPSIA information can be obtained
at www.ICGtesting.com
JSHW012008140824
68134JS00004B/67

9 781681 628714